Clinics in Developmental Medicine No. 146
BEHAVIOURAL APPROACHES
TO PROBLEMS IN CHILDHOOD

© 1998 Mac Keith Press
High Holborn House, 52–54 High Holborn, London WC1V 6RL

Senior Editor: Martin C.O. Bax
Editor: Hilary M. Hart
Managing Editor: Michael Pountney
Sub Editor: Pat Chappelle

Set in Times and Avant Garde on QuarkXPress

The views and opinions expressed herein are those of the authors and do not necessarily
represent those of the publisher

Accuracy of referencing is the responsibility of the authors

First published in this edition 1998

British Library Cataloguing-in-Publication data:
A catalogue record for this book is available from the British Library

ISSN: 0069 4835
ISBN: 1 898683 12 3

Printed by The Lavenham Press Ltd, Water Street, Lavenham, Suffolk
Mac Keith Press is supported by Scope (formerly The Spastics Society)

Clinics in Developmental Medicine No. 146

Behavioural Approaches to Problems in Childhood

Edited by

PATRICIA HOWLIN
Department of Psychology
St George's Medical School
London

1998
Mac Keith Press

Distributed by 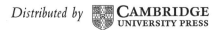 **CAMBRIDGE**
UNIVERSITY PRESS

CONTRIBUTORS

Janet Carr — *Formerly* Regional Tutor in the Psychology of Learning Disability, St George's Hospital Medical School, London, England

Ann N. Garfinkle — Research Assistant, Experimental Education Unit, University of Washington, Seattle, WA, USA

Maryke Groenveld — Psychologist, Psychology Department, BC's Children's Hospital, Vancouver, Canada

James Harris — Professor of Psychiatry and Behavioral Sciences, Pediatrics and Mental Hygiene, Johns Hopkins University School of Medicine, Baltimore, MD, USA

Patricia Howlin — Professor of Clinical Psychology, Department of Psychology, St George's Hospital Medical School, London, England

Gail Joseph — Teacher, Experimental Education Unit, University of Washington, Seattle, WA, USA

Bonnie J. McBride — Project Coordinator, Experimental Education Unit, University of Washington, Seattle, WA, USA

Ilene S. Schwartz — Associate Professor, Experimental Education Unit, University of Washington, Seattle, WA, USA

Stephen Scott — Senior Lecturer and Consultant, Department of Child and Adolescent Psychiatry, Institute of Psychiatry, London, England

Jody Warner-Rogers — Clinical Psychologist, Children's Department, Maudsley Hospital, London, England

CONTENTS

PREFACE   *page vii*

1. CONDUCT DISORDERS   1
   Stephen Scott

2. ATTENTION DEFICIT–HYPERACTIVITY DISORDER   28
   Jody Warner-Rogers

3. AUTISM   54
   Patricia Howlin

4. LEARNING DISABILITIES   78
   Janet Carr

5. COMMUNICATION AND LANGUAGE DISORDERS   95
   Ilene S. Schwartz, Ann N. Garfinkle, Gail Joseph and
   Bonnie J. McBride

6. SENSORY DIFFICULTIES   114
   Maryke Groenveld

7. CEREBRAL PALSY   136
   James Harris

INDEX   152

PREFACE

Developmental disorders in children can take many different forms, affecting their physical development, visual and auditory perception, behaviour and attention, and language and cognitive skills. Often, too, impairments may occur in several of these areas together. Moreover, in all of these conditions the disorder usually covers a wide spectrum of abilities and deficits. To take the case of autism, children may be of above-average IQ or profoundly mentally impaired; they may be entirely nonverbal or possess an apparently sophisticated vocabulary; they may be aloof and withdrawn or over-friendly and socially indiscriminating; and stereotyped behaviours may range from a *potentially* useful preoccupation with dates or maps to simply tearing up bits of paper for hours on end. Similarly, in conditions such as cerebral palsy or visual impairment, not only does the type and extent of the physical or sensory impairment differ from child to child, but problems of language, cognition and behaviour are also likely to be found in varying degrees. Any effective intervention programme, therefore, must be able to take account of both the underlying disorder and also the range and severity of associated or secondary problems. When it comes to devising appropriate intervention strategies there can be no simple solutions. Despite the intrinsic appeal of treatment 'packages' with manuals, videos, set task structures and checklists, the complexity of these disorders means that, at the very best, programmes of this type can only ever be used as *part* of the intervention process. The way in which they are utilized, and approaches to therapy generally, must be adapted, not only to the underlying condition and any associated difficulties, but also to the personality of the individual child, to circumstances and relationships within the family, and to the environments in which interventions take place. Any treatments that claim to work for all children with a particular condition need to be viewed with great scepticism (*e.g.* 'conductive education' for children with cerebral palsy or autism—Delacato 1974, Cummins 1988). The same is true of therapies that are said to remedy a whole range of very different disorders, as was the case with holding therapy (claimed to be equally effective for autism, motor clumsiness, sibling rivalry, childhood depression and a host of other problems—see Welch 1988).

Whilst the focus of the present book is on behaviourally *based* therapy, it is important to be aware of the wide breadth of such methods and to appreciate how far approaches of this kind have advanced since they first began to be used for clinical purposes. A review of the contents of the *Journal of Applied Behaviour Analysis* (which has always contained a significant proportion of child-related articles) over the last three decades helps to emphasize this point. In the first issue (1968) the contents included articles on using sweets or attention to increase verbalizations or the use of adjectives or morphemes in children's speech; the use of electric shocks to reduce aggressive or self-stimulatory behaviours (including rocking) in children with autism and severe learning disabilities; and token programmes to increase 'on-task' behaviours in the classroom or to decrease disruptive behaviours in 'delinquent' boys in residential settings (using access to family visits as one form of back-up reward!). The most sophisticated piece of technology described is a wrist counter for recording the frequency of specific behaviours.

In the last complete issue (1997), major foci are on means of assessing the range and types of reinforcers than may be effective for individuals with severe to profound learning disabilities, the importance of interventions based on functional communication, and the difficulties involved in conducting a functional analysis. Other topics include ways of improving choice and self regulation; programmes to enhance 'happiness' in people with profound learning disabilities; strategies to improve the social interactions between children with autism and their nondisabled peers; environmental modifications to reduce behaviour difficulties; ways of avoiding or defusing problematic situations; and special programmes to encourage children with chronic health problems to adhere to medication regimes. Technology now involves sophisticated hardware that can be used in observational studies, and dedicated software to analyse the interactions and relationships between behaviours. The only slightly disturbing note is the reappearance of articles involving the use of aversive procedures, especially for children showing severe self-injury.

It is hoped that the chapters in this book reflect the many different approaches with an underlying behavioural basis that can be used in intervention. Each of these approaches will need to be modified according to the requirements of the individual child and her/his family. As noted by Owens and MacKinnon (1993), behaviour therapy is not as easy as ABC—even when ABC is translated into *Antecedents*, *Behaviour* and *Consequences*. For many years this tended to be the basic approach to the analysis of problems: first define the behaviour to be addressed, then identify the events that precede it and the consequences that follow and, presumably, reinforce it. However, even defining the behaviour to be worked on may be a relatively complex task, especially when different caretakers, with different priorities, are involved. Identifying antecedents poses many more difficulties. Simply because an event immediately procedes the behaviour in question does not mean that it necessarily has any influence on that behaviour. For a child who processes incoming information more slowly, because of cognitive, linguistic, sensory or attentional difficulties, the perceived relationship between events and behaviour may be very different. Identifying the true consequences of behaviour, again as perceived by the child, may also be fraught with difficulties. Then there is the problem of choosing effective reinforcers. While praise and attention were the mainstay of many early behavioural programmes, it is clear that for some children, especially if they have autism or severe learning disabilities, such consequences may actually be quite aversive. Moreover, a reinforcer that works well under one set of conditions may be totally ineffective in other circumstances. The use of aversives is a further source of contention. In a backlash against the use of aversive consequences (including electric shock, the administration of noxious substances, slapping, shouting, and restitution procedures) the 'Gentle Teaching' movement led to a call for the banning of all aversive strategies, including 'Time Out' (McGee *et al.* 1987). It is easy to understand how the regular use of even fairly mild punitive procedures can eventually lead to abuse (Howlin and Clements 1995). Nevertheless, insistence that no aversive consequences should ever be applied can result in suitable placements breaking down if no sanctions are available to control very disruptive or dangerous behaviours.

It is because of the complexity of issues such as these, that the *ABC* notation in the present book takes on rather a different meaning. The fact that, in most chapters, the description of therapeutic programmes comes well towards the end, is no accident. The emphasis on *Assessment* is deliberate, and crucial. Before any treatment is even considered it is essential to have a full understanding of the particular condition described, to obtain detailed information on all relevant aspects of the child's functioning, to recognize the role that underlying deficits may play in the manifestation of behaviour problems, and to investigate wider aspects of family functioning, and the child's overall quality of life. Only then is it possible to gain a real understanding of the *Breadth* of the problems involved and to develop, in turn, effective and *Comprehensive* strategies that take account of all these factors.

The various chapters also indicate how behaviourally based approaches are rarely, if ever, the only form of intervention required. Attention to family and educational factors is likely to be crucial for long-term outcome. In some instances, too, medically based treatments, including pharmacology, prosthetic devices and physical therapy, may be required. And, although clearly a more difficult goal to attain, improvements in society's understanding of the different conditions will be needed if integration is ever to become a real option.

The principal aim of the book is to reflect the complexity of the different conditions, while at the same time offering practical advice on the strategies that may be utilized by practitioners in order to enhance children's functioning and to minimize potential problems. Behaviourally based procedures have advanced dramatically since they first became routinely used in the early to mid-1960s, and it is to be hoped that the sensitive, and sensible, use of such strategies may have a major impact on the lives of children with developmental problems and all those who work with or care for them.

PATRICIA HOWLIN

REFERENCES

Cummins, R.A. (1988) *The Neurologically Impaired Child: Doman–Delacato Techniques Reappraised.* London: Croom Helm.

Delacato, C.H. (1974) *The Ultimate Stranger: The Autistic Child.* New York: Doubleday.

Howlin, P., Clements, J. (1995) 'Is it possible to assess the impact of abuse on children with pervasive developmental disorders?' *Journal of Autism and Developmental Disorders,* **25**, 1–17.

McGee, J.J., Menolascino, P.E., Hobbs, D.C., Menousek, P.E. (1987) *Gentle Teaching: A Non-Aversive Approach to Helping Persons with Mental Retardation.* New York: Human Science Press.

Owens, R.G., MacKinnon, S. (1993) 'The functional analysis of challenging behaviours: some conceptual and theoretical problems.' *In:* Jones, R.S.P., Eayrs, C.B. (Eds.) *Challenging Behaviour and Intellectual Disability: a Psychological Perspective.* Clevedon, Avon: BILD Publications, pp. 224–239.

Welch, M. (1988) *Holding Time.* London: Century Hutchinson.

1
CONDUCT DISORDER

Stephen Scott

'Conduct disorder' is a term used to denote a syndrome of core symptoms characterized by the *persistent failure to control behaviour appropriately within socially defined rules*. According to most epidemiological studies, it is the commonest child psychiatric problem. It is often persistent, has a heavy cost for society, and yet has proved to be largely untreatable. Conduct problems involve three overlapping domains of behaviour: *defiance* of the will of someone in authority, *aggressiveness*, and *antisocial behaviour* that violates other people's rights, property or person. None of these is in itself abnormal or pathological, and indeed there are occasions when one tries to promote some of these behaviours in overdependent children. Disobedient and destructive behaviour is a part of normal development that usually diminishes with maturity, and a diagnosis of conduct disorder should be made only when the behaviours are both extreme and persistent.

Presentation

The manifestations change with age. Younger children are more likely to show the signs of 'oppositional defiant disorder' which is a subtype of conduct disorder in the World Health Organization's classification system, ICD-10 (WHO 1993), but a separate condition in the American DSM-IV (American Psychiatric Association 1994). The criterion behaviours for oppositional defiant disorder (Table 1.1) should occur "considerably more frequently than in other children of the same mental age". The DSM-IV criteria for conduct disorder (Table 1.2) are more likely to be met by older children, and are closer to those for adult antisocial personality disorder. This definition is less likely to include girls than previous definitions since early sexual experience, early substance abuse and chronic violation of rules have been dropped. Henceforward in this chapter the term conduct disorder will be used irrespective of age.

COMMON ASSOCIATED FEATURES
Psychiatric symptoms
• *Hyperactivity*. Restlessness, inattentiveness, impulsiveness and general overactivity often coexist, and this combination makes the outcome worse.

• *Emotional symptoms*. About a third of affected subjects show significant emotional symptoms, most commonly unhappiness and misery. Whether this should be seen as a separate comorbid condition or as part of the general underlying distress is debated; it does

TABLE 1.1
DSM-IV criteria for oppositional–defiant disorder*

Disturbance for six months with at least four of the following:

(1) Often loses temper	(5) Often shifts blame to others
(2) Often argues with adults	(6) Often touchy or easily annoyed
(3) Often defies adult requests or rules	(7) Often angry and resentful
(4) Often deliberately annoys others	(8) Often spiteful or vindictive*

*American Psychiatric Association (1994).

TABLE 1.2
DSM-IV criteria for conduct disorder*

Disturbance for 12 months involving at least three of the following:

(1) Often bullies, threatens or intimidates	(9) Has destroyed other's property
(2) Often starts fights	(10) Has broken into car or house
(3) Has used serious weapons in fights	(11) Cons others
(4) Physically cruel to people	(12) Stealing without force
(5) Physically cruel to animals	(13) Often out at night without permission
(6) Stealing with force	(14) Ran away from home overnight twice
(7) Has forced someone into sexual acts	(15) Often truants, beginning under 13 years
(8) Fire setting to cause damage	

*American Psychiatric Association (1994).

not seem to lead to a better or worse outcome in terms of conduct disorder, and neither is it clearly a risk factor for adult depression.

Scholastic failure
Many subjects have poor achievements in terms of grades and level of work, often demonstrating specific learning deficits. On testing, a third of children with conduct disorder have specific reading disorder, defined as being more than two standard deviations below the reading level expected for their age and intelligence (Rutter and Yule 1975, Hinshaw 1992, Mandel 1997). Conversely, a third of children with specific reading disorder have conduct disorder. This association could be due to any of three possibilities. Firstly, disruptive behaviour may interfere with classroom learning. Secondly, children who do not have the ability to understand and participate in class may become frustrated and disruptive as a result. Thirdly, both disruptiveness and reading problems may stem from a third factor such as hyperactivity. Different mechanisms seem to be at work in different children. For a substantial proportion, there is good evidence that specific learning difficulties were present from an early age, *e.g.* the child had delayed language acquisition. Lower IQ is associated with conduct disorder but probably not as strongly as poor achievement.

Impaired social relationships
Disruptive children often become unpopular with their peers and frequently have no enduring friends. They commonly show poor social skills with both peers and adults, *e.g.* they have difficulty sustaining a game or promoting positive social interchanges. Poor peer relation-

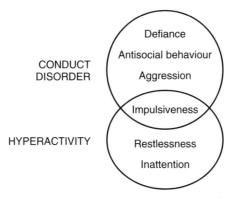

Fig. 1.1. The overlap of symptoms of conduct disorder and hyperactivity.

ships predict unfavourable outcome. ICD-10 divides conduct disorder into 'unsocialized' and 'socialized' types according to whether the young person has normal peer relationships or not; DSM-IV has no comparable categories. In clinical practice, the great majority of children with conduct disorder do have impaired peer relationships. Nevertheless, there is limited evidence from cluster analytic studies for a relatively small group of conduct-disordered youngsters who do make enduring friendships, display altruistic behaviour, feel guilt or remorse, refrain from blaming others, and show concern for others. These individuals with socialized conduct disorder tend to be older and to engage in less aggressive antisocial acts such as stealing, truanting and drinking alcohol. They could be considered 'well-adjusted juvenile delinquents' who are not regarded as deviant within their own subculture.

DIFFERENTIAL DIAGNOSIS
There is usually not much doubt about the diagnosis if detailed information is obtained from more than one source. Multiple informants are vital since conduct problems may occur in only one setting, *e.g.* just at home or just at school. Epidemiological studies have shown that there is fairly low correlation between teacher and parent ratings of conduct problems.

Differential diagnoses to consider include:

(1) *Adjustment reaction to external stressor.* This can be diagnosed when onset occurs soon after exposure to an identifiable psychosocial stressor such as divorce, bereavement, adoption, trauma or abuse—within one month according to ICD-10 and within three months according to DSM-IV—and when symptoms do not persist for more than six months after the cessation of the stress or its consequences.

(2) *Attention deficit–hyperactivity disorder (ADHD)/hyperactivity.* Conduct disorder can be mistaken for ADHD/hyperactivity and vice versa. This is partly due to overlap in symptoms, as shown in Figure 1.1. Defiance, aggression and intentionally antisocial behaviour are not part of pure hyperactivity. In clinically referred populations, conduct disorder and hyperactivity often coexist, and this can result in the hyperactivity itself being missed. Hyperactivity is discussed in Chapter 2.

3

(3) *No disorder.* The child's behaviour is within the normal range, but parents or teachers have unrealistically high expectations.

(4) *Subcultural deviance.* Some youngsters are antisocial but not particularly aggressive or defiant, and they are well adjusted within a deviant peer culture that approves of recreational drug use, shoplifting, etc. They could be assigned an ICD-10 diagnosis of socialized conduct disorder, but it is arguably a mistake to pathologize what can be seen as a cultural variant.

(5) *Autistic spectrum disorders.* These are often accompanied by marked tantrums or destructiveness, and these conduct problems are occasionally the principal cause for referral Asking about the other symptoms of autistic-spectrum disorders will reveal their presence (see Chapter 3).

PREVALENCE
Conduct disorder has been diagnosed in 4–10 per cent of children, according to the criteria used and the area studied (Rutter *et al.* 1975, Kazdin 1995). The prevalence is particularly high in deprived inner-city areas. Boys are conduct disordered around three times more commonly than girls. The age of onset can vary considerably, but in persistent cases has usually begun around 3–6 years of age. Conduct disorder is associated with lower socio-economic status (this covers a multitude of variables) and large family size.

Aetiology
NATURE OR NURTURE?
Although conduct disorder commonly clusters in families, behavioural genetics studies indicate that shared family environment is more important than shared genes. Thus, although twin studies have shown a high concordance for monozygotic pairs at around 70–80 per cent, the concordance for dizygotic pairs is also high at around 60–70 per cent, suggesting a limited genetic component (DiLalla and Gottesman 1989). Adoption studies have shown the influence of the biological parents is important, but somewhat less so than that of the adoptive ones. What is particularly damaging is the combination of a genetic predisposition (as indexed for example by a criminal father or either birth parent being alcoholic) plus an adverse upbringing, as shown in Figure 1.2 (Bohman 1996).

Genetic influences seem to play a stronger role in the development of adult antisocial personality and criminality than in childhood antisocial behaviour and conduct problems. Cytogenetic and molecular genetics studies have added little so far; epidemiological studies do not suggest a particular association with the XYY karyotype once the effect of low IQ has been allowed for.

FAMILY ENVIRONMENT
Parent–child interaction patterns
Fine-grained analysis by Patterson (1982) has shown that the moment-to-moment responses of parents towards children have a powerful effect on their behaviour. In families where there is a child with conduct disorder, the children typically get ignored when they are behaving reasonably, but are criticized and shouted at when they misbehave. The consequence

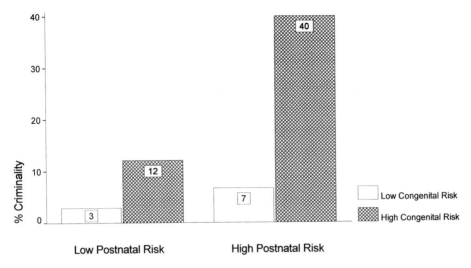

Fig. 1.2. Antisocial behaviour in adoptees: criminality rates in youths adopted as infants. (Data from Bohman 1996.)

is that to gain attention, they have to behave badly. What is perhaps surprising is that they prefer negative attention to none at all, and are prepared to elicit often unpleasant and frankly painful reactions from their parents. By contrast, children who receive a reasonable amount of positive attention within the family tend not to behave in a way which elicits negative attention. All this can be summarized as the 'attention rule', which states that children will behave in whatever way necessary to gain a reasonable amount of attention.

Other behaviours by parents can unwittingly raise the probability of disruptive behaviour in the child. Giving up insisting something unpleasant is carried out (*e.g.* tidying up the toys) unintentionally rewards the child for whining and refusing to do it, thus making whining and refusing more likely next time a request is made. Giving in to demands for something pleasant (*e.g.* sweets) has the same effects.

To date, most emphasis in social learning theory has been on the harmful effect of negative behaviour. However, research by Gardner (1987) has made it clear that the presence of positive parental behaviour is equally important. Children with antisocial behaviour are ignored for a lot of the time by their parents, who do not respond to their overtures to join in activities, nor praise them when they are behaving well. Not only does this make quiet activity less likely since no attention is forthcoming, but no models are provided for the child to learn social skills such as turn-taking, negotiating skills and so forth.

The implications of the power of the interaction patterns are far-reaching. Rather than construing the child as innately aggressive or with an antisocial type of personality which is unchangeable, the child can be seen as responding to the immediate context s/he is in. Change the context, and you will change the behaviour of the child. This can occur over minutes or hours. It allows some therapeutic optimism, since if the response contingencies around the child are altered, improvement can occur.

Parenting practices
Conduct disorder is strongly associated with harsh, erratic discipline, hostility directed at the child, lack of warmth, and poor supervision (Farrington 1994). Follow-up and intervention studies show clearly that these factors have a causal role in initiating and maintaining the child's disorder, and are not simply a reaction to the child's behaviour. Discord between parents is also associated with antisocial behaviour, especially persistent conduct disorder (Richman *et al.* 1982).

Psychiatric disorder in parents
Depression features commonly in mothers; alcoholism, drug abuse and psychoses are seen not infrequently in either parent. This is an important influence, but in childhood its effect is exerted mainly through the quality of interaction and parenting practices and is not specific to any particular psychiatric condition in the parents (Rutter and Quinton 1984).

Criminality of father
As an environmental influence, this is important (it was one of the family adversities coded in the adoption study depicted in Figure 1.2) and may be mediated through parent–child interactions and parenting practices as described above, plus an antisocial set of values and living in a deprived neighbourhood.

Sexual abuse
Sexual abuse can lead to the emergence of conduct problems in girls or boys who were previously free of such problems.

ENVIRONMENT BEYOND THE FAMILY
School factors
School factors have been shown to affect conduct disorder rates independently of home background: poorly-organized, unfriendly schools with low staff morale, high staff turnover and poor contact with parents have higher conduct disorder rates even when catchment area characteristics have been allowed for (Rutter *et al.* 1979).

Peer influences
Peer influences have also been shown to affect conduct problems independently. Conduct disorder is more likely in children who associate with friends who have an antisocial attitude, value aggression, and commit destructive and rule-breaking acts (Dishion *et al.* 1994).

Neighbourhood
Conduct problems are associated with overcrowding, poor housing, and poor neighbourhoods. How much these factors are causal or simply markers for other family or socioeconomic variables is unclear. However, it is plausible that stressful living conditions with few amenities for children and many other demands on parents impair their ability to bring up their children constructively and responsively.

CHILD CHARACTERISTICS

Constitution, temperament and personality
Characteristics proposed as implicated in conduct disorder have included neurotransmitter imbalance, hormonal excess (notably testosterone), metabolic variations such as low cholesterol, and abnormal arousal patterns with failure to calm down after frustration. None of these show replicable findings of any generality. However, infants with temperaments classified as 'difficult' are more likely to be referred for aggressive problems later on (Thomas *et al.* 1968).

Cognitive processes
Aggressive and challenging behaviour is far commoner in children and young people with learning disabilities (Scott 1994). Significant cognitive attributional bias has been shown in aggressive children whereby they are more likely to perceive neutral acts by others as hostile. As the child gets more disliked and rejected by her/his peers, the opportunity for seeing things this way increases (Dodge and Lochman 1994). Social skills are lacking. Emotional processes in conduct disordered children have been little studied, although self-esteem is often low and coexistent misery common. The role of academic achievement is discussed above.

Assessment of the child
The greater part of the history will usually be taken from the mother, sometimes with the father or another relative or friend present. Only aspects of the psychiatric history specific to conduct disorder are described here. For details of the remainder of the psychiatric history which should be taken, the reader should consult one of the main introductory texts, *e.g.* Goodman and Scott (1997). In addition to speaking to the parent, it is vital to speak to the child alone and also to contact the school.

Conduct symptoms
The severity and frequency of defiant, aggressive and antisocial acts in the last month or so should be established in detail—some parents are prone to catalogue all 'bad' things done over the last year or even since birth. Attention and activity should be enquired about in the same detailed way (see Chapter 2), since hyperactivity is a common and easily over-looked accompaniment of conduct problems (see Figure 1.1). Though it is worth enquiring about impulsiveness, this could be part of either hyperactivity or conduct problems. One should not forget to enquire about emotional symptoms, particularly unhappiness and misery. Part of the problem may derive from things that are upsetting the child, *e.g.* a father who often fails to turn up for his access visits, or a mother who never seems to appreciate the child however hard s/he tries. The strength of these concerns may only come out in an individual interview with the child, and could easily be missed if the family are only ever seen together.

Seeing the child alone
Seeing the child alone at some stage allows one to ask about what is going on in the family

and can be very revealing. Children (like adults) almost always appreciate having their views heard, and this will increase the chance that they will want to come back. There may be quite punitive practices going on which the child would not have discussed in front of her/his parent/s. Sometimes a child will reveal details about the family which are directly relevant, *e.g.* father's drinking, imminent separation of the parents, etc. At other times marked emotional symptoms will be revealed (see below) which may include worries about an ill member of the family dying, the reexperiencing of some trauma minimized by the parents (*e.g.* a car crash without serious injuries). Asking a child why s/he behaves that way will seldom be fruitful, usually eliciting the answer "don't know" as most children genuinely are unaware why.

Physical examination
This should be carried out in all cases. It need not take more than five to ten minutes, and should cover height, weight and head circumference; a short neurological examination; and examination of facies, hands and feet for dysmorphic features. In the author's clinic 10–20 per cent of affected children have shown positive findings, which have included several dysmorphic syndromes.

Information from school
A school report is essential, covering antisocial behaviour, ability to concentrate and sit still, peer relations, and scholastic attainments, including any test results. There are occasions when troublesome behaviour in class can take up so much of the teacher's time that significant reading difficulties can be overlooked or simply regarded as a consequence of the bad behaviour.

If hyperactivity seems likely, then a standardized questionnaire such as the Strengths and Difficulties Questionnaire (SDQ—Goodman 1997) filled in by the teacher is helpful in determining the extent to which the symptoms are present at school as well as at home. There are longer questionnaires with more items covering hyperactivity such as those devised by Conners (Goyette *et al.* 1978) and by Achenbach (1991), but they take up more teacher time and do not appear to add any greater specificity than short ones (Goodman and Scott 1998). If hyperactivity is present in both contexts and is severe, medication may be warranted. Whilst medication is unhelpful for conduct symptoms alone, where there is coexistent hyperactivity it may reduce aggression considerably.

Where the child is failing academically, getting an intelligence test and a reading test done can be invaluable in pinpointing learning difficulties. It is not unusual for a child labelled as only naughty to turn out to have severe specific reading difficulties (dyslexia) or even mild generalized learning disability (mental retardation).

Assessment of parenting
HISTORY AND EXAMINATION
Parenting practices should be enquired about in detail, with a blow-by-blow account of what happened before, during and after a recent episode of troublesome behaviour. Who 'won' the encounter? What was said? How long did it take for relations to return to normal? More

generally, it is useful to ask how much praise and encouragement is given for constructive behaviour, and how much time is spent in joint activities. One should try to gauge the parents' sensitivity to the child's moods and needs, and how much they take these into account when negotiating conflicts and planning the child's life.

The parents' emotional tone and attitude towards the child should be considered. Asking about the child's good qualities can be helpful. Is there some warmth and approval despite the child's difficulties, or is the tone entirely negative? Powerful beliefs may be discovered which will need to be addressed if treatment is to progress, *e.g.* "There's something wrong in his head", or "He's just like his father. He was rotten too."

Direct observation of parents and children is invaluable in getting a picture of their interactions, albeit in atypical circumstances. Are clear boundaries set, or is the child allowed to get away with almost anything? For example, how do the parents react when the child tries to leave the room? Is good behaviour praised or ignored? Is the child handled sensitively?

DIMENSIONS OF PARENTING

When assessing the quality of parenting, and planning intervention, the following dimensions are useful to bear in mind:

• *Boundaries.* Are appropriate house rules set and enforced? For instance, is there a regular routine? Are there clear expectations about, say, not fighting with other children?

• *Supervision.* Does the parent know exactly where and with whom their child is, through-out the day? (or is s/he free to go off truanting, or to go playing on an estate getting into trouble with other poorly supervised children?) For younger children, are they in direct sight? (Or are they upstairs, risking accidental injury with medicines, hot water, glass, etc.?)

• *Discipline.* Are expectations for what is reasonable behaviour realistic given the child's age? What happens when the child disobeys? Do the parents deploy a range of strategies in a consistent way? Do they give clear commands and then follow through with a consequence if it is not complied with? Is there a flexible range of strategies, from ignoring minor infringements to withdrawal of privileges to being sent to a boring room? Or is there a string of weakly couched commands with no consequences, until several minutes later there is an exasperated angry explosion of uncontrolled parental wrath leading to wounding words, sometimes with wounding actions too? Do both parents agree and support each other, or are they inconsistent so that the child has two sets of rules to contend with?

• *Emotional attunement and availability.* Is the parent reliably and predictably open and affectionate, available and sensitive to the child's needs? Is the way open for the child to become securely attached to the parent?

• *Positive involvement and stimulation.* How often do the parents play with the child? How often do they organize an activity for the child, such as swimming or a walk to the park? How often is the child praised, and what encouragement is given for achievements, however small, to foster a sense of pride and self-worth? (This may range from very little in neglectful families where perhaps the child is stuck in front of the TV for many hours a day, to high involvement but of a very critical kind by an unrealistically overambitious parent who, for example, is forever trying to teach the child, who contrarily may end up feeling stupid.

• *Ability to put the child's needs first.* Can the parents organize themselves to meet the child's needs, or do they put themselves first, *e.g.* by going out in the evenings to have fun while leaving the child with unsuitable adults, or taking excessive drugs or alcohol so that the child's needs are neglected for several hours?

• *Physical care.* Is the child well fed, reasonably dressed, and generally looked after? Has s/he been taken to the doctor for appointments where indicated? Is s/he growing adequately?

SOME PARENTING PATTERNS REVEALED BY ASSESSMENT
Every family is different and the particular mix of personalities and predicaments is unique. Nonetheless, some patterns emerge regularly, which may be seen singly, or in combination:
(i) Neglect of child, with poor physical care, low level of involvement, lack of supervision, and little awareness of child's emotional needs.
(ii) Rejection of child, with chronic lack of warmth, punitive harsh discipline, blame and scapegoating, yet often adequate physical conditions and reasonable treatment of other children in the family (Reid *et al.* 1987, McGee and Wolfe 1991, Cicchetti and Lynch 1993).
(iii) Episodic neglect or abuse, interspersed with spells of reasonable parenting, due for example to alcoholism, or a parent under stress with no support.
(iv) Emotional overinvolvement, with inability to set limits due to fear of upsetting child, and overprotection.
(v) Parenting generally adequate, but insufficient for this child, who has, for instance, a difficult temperament or special needs.
(vi) Parenting normal, parents delivering a reasonable level of care to a child whose difficulties are due not to upbringing but rather to constitutional factors, for example autism or hyperkinesis.

Underlying causes of parenting difficulty
PARENT-RELATED PROBLEMS
• *Experienced a harsh upbringing themselves.* Such parents had a harsh and insensitive upbringing, and were possibly physically or sexually abused, or brought up by a succession of foster parents or in a children's home (Zeanah and Zeanah 1989). Parents like these often have little idea how to look after children. Two groups exist, those who are aware of or can recognize the impact of their own experience and wish to make amends, and those who show no realization that children could be brought up any other way (Spieker and Booth 1988, Lyons-Ruth 1996). This distinction is important as it predicts considerable difference

in the sensitivity of parenting and emotional security of the child's relationship with the parent (Routh *et al.* 1995), as well as the likelihood that treatment will be successful.

• *Unrealistic expectations.* Some parents have a poor idea of what young children can and cannot do (*e.g.* with a 3-year-old, they may expect them to sit still and play unattended for half an hour, or expect them to get dressed without help), and may get cross or abusive when they fail to obey instructions (Azar and Rohrbeck 1986). They may have little idea what motivates children, for example believing that promising a child a bicycle or pet kitten for their next birthday in three months time will act as an effective reward for immediate behaviour, when in the child's mind it is too far ahead. These parents are often young, or have not had any experience of children, *e.g.* never had to look after younger siblings or relatives' children.

• *Difficulties with all relationships.* Here the parent not only has difficulty getting on with the child, but also finds it hard to maintain any lasting close relationships. There may be a pattern of brief and unsatisfactory love relationships, a lack of substantial friends (aside from superficial acquaintances), frequent changes of jobs when employed due to arguments at work, and difficulties negotiating with the wider public, including doctors. Often their view of relationships is dismissive and hopeless (Crittenden 1988).

• *Pervasive belief that the child is bad.* These parents may be reasonably competent in other domains (they may provide excellent care for a sibling), but they have a pervasive belief that this child is no good and so subject her/him to ongoing emotional abuse. For example, a mother might believe that her son is becoming just like his father, who was a violent criminal and hit her; or that right from the unwanted pregnancy onwards he has ruined her life. This can lead to a vicious downward spiral where everything the child does is seen as evil and intended to 'wind up' the mother.

• *Psychiatric disorder.* Depression is particularly common in mothers, and may easily be missed unless directly asked about. Drug and alcohol abuse, and personality difficulties (see above) are also common (Walker *et al.* 1989, Dinwiddie and Bucholz 1993).

• *Limited intellectual capacity.* Low parental IQ can impair several areas of functioning (Downdney and Skuse 1990). This may have been previously undetected and, if suspected, should lead to psychometric testing.

SITUATION-RELATED PROBLEMS
• *Unsupportive partner.* Here one partner (usually the father, but occasionally the mother) is unhelpful and offers little practical or emotional support to the other. Arguments are common and sometimes lead to violence, often witnessed by the child. Frequently there is inconsistency between the parents on how the child is handled (Cicchetti and Hares 1991).

• *Isolation.* Some parents have few friends or relatives with whom to share practical or emotional aspects of childcare. Often, too, they have few places to go out of the house. This kind of parent can be particularly stuck in a destructive relationship with a child, and gains made in parent training are usually lost soon after the programme finishes (Wahler 1980).

• *Material lack.* Poor housing with insufficient space for the child to play in can contribute to parenting difficulty. Debt and other financial difficulties add to the burden, as do poverty and lack of general facilities, *e.g.* washing machine, transport, etc. (Gelles 1992)

• *Other demands.* Some adults cannot give sufficient time and energy as is necessary to the index child because they have other commitments, *e.g.* a job, other children or relatives to look after, etc. (Cicchetti and Lynch 1993).

CHILD-RELATED PROBLEMS
The parenting may be adequate for an easy child, but may have broken down due to the child being very difficult, with other problems additional to the conduct disorder (which can be trying enough in its own right).

• *Behavioural difficulties.* Severe hyperactivity and autistic spectrum disorders can be especially wearing. As mentioned above, some children are born with more difficult temperaments.

• *Generalized learning disability.* This may underlie some of the conduct problems and lead to a far greater burden of care. Fifty per cent of children with an IQ <50 have a psychiatric disorder, most commonly conduct disorder, often described as 'challenging behaviour' in this group (Scott 1994).

• *Abuse.* Undetected sexual or physical abuse outside the family (or with a previous family in fostered or adopted children) may add to the child's disturbance (Crittenden *et al.* 1994, Okun *et al.* 1994).

• *Brain injury.* Preterm children who suffered intraventricular haemorrhages have an increased incidence of behavioural difficulties. There may also be attachment problems for the parents due to the prolonged separation and worry. Postnatal insult such as meningitis or a road traffic accident can lead to personality changes which make a child hard to look after.

• *Physical illness.* Children whose illness requires high levels of care, *e.g.* cystic fibrosis, cerebral palsy, severe eczema, etc., may stress their parents to breaking point.

Behaviourally based parenting programmes
Behaviourally based parenting programmes have repeatedly been shown in well-conducted trials to be an effective treatment for conduct disorder (Kazdin 1997). Specific details of

TABLE 1.3
Contents of a parenting programme

Part 1	*Techniques for increasing desired behaviour:* (a) play (b) praise and rewards
Part 2	*Techniques for reducing unwanted behaviour:* (a) giving clear commands (b) setting consistent consequences for disobedience (c) ignoring (d) 'time out'
Part 3	*Strategies for avoiding trouble:* (a) planning ahead (b) negotiating (c) promoting problem-solving (d) handling common trying situations

their content, evidence of their effectiveness and some common difficulties encountered are described below. After this an overview of other treatments for conduct disorder is given.

CONTENT
Most programmes can be divided into three parts, as shown in Table 1.3. More extensive descriptions are given by Forehand and McMahon (1981) and Barkley (1997).

Part 1. Techniques for increasing desired behaviour
To give a feel for how sessions go, the first two will be described in some detail:

• *First session: Play.* The programme starts with this, perhaps the most fundamental aspect of improving the relationship with the child. Parents are asked to follow the child's lead rather than impose their own ideas. Instead of giving directions, teaching and asking questions during play, parents are instructed simply to describe what the child is doing, to give a running commentary on their child's actions. The target is to give at least four of these 'descriptive comments' per minute. If the parent has difficulty in getting going, the practitioner suggests precisely what they should do, for example by saying "I'd like you to say to Johnny: 'You've put the car in the garage'." As soon as the parent complies, the practitioner gives feedback: "That was a good descriptive comment."

After 10-15 minutes, this directly supervised play ends and the parent is 'debriefed' for half an hour or more alone with the clinician. How the parent felt while doing it is explored, and reservations and difficulties which arose are addressed. Usually the effect of their behaviour on the child during the training session is soon observed by the parent. Typically, the child is seen to settle and spend longer than usual playing purposefully with one game, rather than rushing round the room switching inconsequentially from one activity to another. Misbehaviour is usually at a lower level than normal. Experiencing this close, nonjudgemental attention is surprisingly powerful for children, who at best feel they are 'the apple of their

13

parent's eye'. For parents who have got to a state of affairs where virtually all communication with the child is nagging and complaining, play is an important first step in mending the relationship. It often helps the parent to realize it can be fun together, and to begin to have positive feelings for the child again. Parents are asked to do homework by playing with their child using these techniques for 10 minutes every day.

• *Second session: Checking progress with homework; elaboration of play skills.* For the first 20 minutes, the previous week's 'homework' of playing at home is gone over with the parent in considerable detail. Often there are practical reasons for not doing it ("I have to look after the other children, I've got no help") and parents are then encouraged to solve the problem and find ways around the difficulty (solutions arrived at might include doing the play after the younger sibling has gone to bed; getting the oldest child to look after the baby while the parent plays with the toddler; asking the parent's sister to come in to cover for the 15 minute play time). With other parents there may be emotional blocks ("It feels wrong—no one ever played with me as a child") which need to be overcome before the parent feels able to practice the homework. By going over whatever the difficulty may be and gently pushing for a solution to try out, parents see that the clinician is quietly determined to have the changes implemented. In a way, the parents themselves are testing out the practitioner to see what will happen if they (rather than their child) don't comply with the rules. Getting over the hump of inertia is often very energizing—the parents feel better for getting something done.

After this, the live session with the child is carried out. Usually this continues where the previous one left off, and further develops the parent's play skills. This time the parent is encouraged to go beyond describing the child's behaviour and to make comments describing the child's likely mood state, *e.g.* "You're really trying hard making that tower", or "That puzzle is making you really fed up". This process has benefits for both the parent and the child. The parent gets better at observing the fine details of the child's behaviour and this makes them more sensitive to the child's mood. This ability is important if responsive parenting is to develop, and is poorly developed in unskilled parents (Wahler and Sansbury 1990); thus the problem is a perceptual one as well as a lack of skills. The child feels appreciated for what s/he is doing, and knows her/his efforts and disappointments are appreciated. Through this process s/he gradually gets better at understanding and labelling her/his own emotional states, a crucial step in gaining self-control in frustrating situations. A feature of out-of-control children brought up in insensitive parenting environments is their inability to describe their emotions, often at the most basic level (so-called 'alexithymia') (Berenbaum 1996).

• *Subsequent sessions.* These follow the same pattern of: (1) reviewing the previous week's homework, (2) direct training of interaction with the child, and (3) discussion afterwards of how it went. The speed at which the content is covered depends on progress. Later sessions build on an ethic of *praise and rewards*. A motto for this part of the programme is 'catch them being good' and then praise them. Empirical studies show that in families where parents are having difficulty controlling their children, when the child does behave

14

sociably, s/he is ignored (Patterson 1982). As a consequence, the only way for the child to gain attention is through being naughty. This leads to a situation where the parent is unwittingly actively training up their child to be antisocial. To reverse this state of affairs requires the parents to praise their child for lots of mundane, everyday behaviours such as playing quietly on their own, eating nicely, getting dressed the first time they are asked, and so on. In this way the frequency of desired behaviour increases. However, many parents find this difficult. Firstly, they may say "but he *should* be doing these things anyway, without being praised for it—there's really no need." Secondly, when their child has mis-behaved earlier in the day they are still cross, and this prevents them praising good behaviour when it occurs. Thirdly, some parents find that even when they want to praise their child, the whole process feels alien to them. Often they never experienced praise themselves as a child. In this situation, direct one-to-one intervention is invaluable, as the clinician can rehearse with the parent precisely how to speak to the child. Usually with practice it becomes easier.

Part 2. Techniques for reducing unwanted behaviour
• *Commands.* A hallmark of ineffective parenting is a continuing stream of ineffectual, nagging demands for the child to do something. In the programme, parents are taught to reduce the number of commands, but to make them much more authoritative. This is done through altering both the manner in which they are given, and what is said. The manner should be forceful (not sitting down, timidly requesting from the other end of the room; instead, standing over the child, fixing her/him in the eye, and in a clear firm voice giving the instruction). The emotional tone should be calm, without shouting and criticism. The content should be phrased directly ("I want you to . .") and not indirectly or as a question ("Wouldn't you like to . ."). It should be specific, labelling the desired behaviour which the child can understand, so it is clear to her/him when s/he has complied ("Keep the sand in the box") rather than vague ("Do be tidy"). It should be simple (one action at a time, not a chain of orders), and performable immediately. Commands should be phrased as what the parent *does* want the child to do, not as what s/he should *stop* doing ("Please speak quietly" rather than "Stop shouting"). If a child is in the middle of an activity, then rather than abruptly ordering a stop, a warning should be given ("In two minutes you'll have to go to bed"). Rather than threatening the child with vague, dire consequences ("You're going to be sorry you did that"), *when–then* commands should be given ("When you've laid the table, then you can watch TV").

• *Consequences for disobedience.* Consequences for disobedience should be applied as soon as possible. They must always be followed through—children quickly learn to cal-culate the probability they will be applied, and if in fact a sanction is only given every third occasion, a child is being taught that s/he can misbehave the rest of the time. Simple logical consequences should be devised and enforced for everyday situations, *e.g.* if water is splashed out of the bath, the bath will end; if a child refuses to eat dinner, there will be no pudding. The consequences should 'fit the crime', should not be punitive, and should not be long-term (no bike riding for a month), as this will lead to a sense of hopelessness in the child who may see no point in behaving well if it seems there is nothing to gain. Planning ahead and giving the child a warning enables them to have an element of choice in their behaviour, and teaches them they have a measure of control over the situation ("If you haven't picked up the toys by 7 o'clock, there'll be no snack or story"). Consistency of enforcement is central.

• *Ignore and distract.* This sounds easy but is a hard skill to teach parents. Whining, arguing, swearing and tantrums are not dangerous to children or to other people and can usually safely be ignored. The technique is very effective when applied. Children soon realize they are getting no payoff for the behaviours and soon stop. Vice-versa, if acting this way gets them attention and shows them they can annoy and 'wind up' their parents, they will continue to hone their skills in so doing. Ignoring means avoiding discussion, avoiding eye contact and turning away, but staying in the room to monitor. As soon as the child begins to behave appropriately, it is essential to attend and give praise. This is central to shaping desirable behaviour—ignoring will only reduce undesirable behaviour, which is not the same thing. Many parents find this difficult as they are often still angry with the child. Distraction is useful with 2- to 4-year-olds—after ignoring for some moments, an interesting alternative activity likely to capture the child's imagination is offered.

• *Time out.* The full name of this is 'time out from positive reinforcement', and as pointed out in Chapter 4, it can take many different forms. One method is to put the child in some place away from a reasonably pleasant context. This will not be the case if the home is generally negative, when being sent to a room alone will be a relief and not a punishment. Equally, if the room has lots of interesting toys the same will apply. Time out should be in a boring place (end of the corridor, porch, toilet, etc.) for a previously agreed reason (hitting, breaking things, etc.—not minor infringements) for a short time (say one minute for each year of age). However, the child must be quiet for the last minute—if s/he is still screaming, s/he stays in for as long as it takes until s/he has been quiet for a minute. For the first few times, this may be for 30–40 minutes or more as the child tests out the new system. However, soon the period will reduce to a few minutes only. Parents must resist responding to taunts and cries from the child during time out, as this will reinforce the child by giving attention. Time out also provides a break for the adult to calm down. At the end of the period, the child has served the punishment and should not be scolded. If the reason for the time out was failure to carry out an instruction, the instruction should be given again (otherwise the child is being taught that by disobeying s/he can avoid complying). Time out should not need to be used more than a few times a week. If the child is spending more than about two hours per week in time out, something is going wrong and the situation needs investigating. Most children are sent there for only a few minutes a week or not at all—the knowledge that it is there is often enough to help the child comply (White *et al.* 1972, Scarboro and Forehand 1975, Gardner *et al.* 1976, Hobbs *et al.* 1978, Herbert 1987, Barkley 1997).

Part 3. Strategies for avoiding trouble
• *Planning ahead.* Parents are taught to keep a diary of when problem behaviours occurred,

what led up to them, and what happened after (the 'ABC' of behaviour: *A*ntecedents, *B*ehaviour, *C*onsequences). They learn from this that tantrums do not occur randomly (though they used to seem that way), but that there are certain high-risk situations and times. They learn to recognize their own role after the event in reinforcing the bad behaviour. By rearranging the child's schedule, many difficult situations can be avoided. A grandmother can look after the child during supermarket trips, a shower can be substituted for a bath, long phone calls to friends can be made in the evening, and so on.

• *Negotiating.* It is surprising how many parents are ignorant of their children's fears and main desires, as well as their expectations in everyday situations. The children are seen as difficult because they won't fit in and do as they're told. However, often in fact they are subject to a bewildering flow of unreasonable demands and are frustratingly cut short without warning when they are quietly enjoying an activity. Getting parents to stop and listen to their children's wishes and fears is often a revelation for them. Then, planning how to accommodate the child's wishes while fitting in with the family goals for the day is practised. For the child, having been consulted about the plan and contributing to it usually leads them to behave more calmly and contentedly.

• *Developing a problem-solving approach with the child.* This is another strategy which helps stop impulsive reactions to frustration in children and helps them slow down and devise their own solutions. Over the longer term this promotes independence. There are programmes of this kind taught directly by professionals to children (Petersen and Gannoni 1992), but one can also get the parents to use the process with their children. This has the advantage of getting the parents to think this way too. *Step 1* involves stopping to hear the child's side of the story. For *Step 2*, the child is encouraged to generate as many solutions as possible to the problem, however silly (*e.g.* "hit him/take his toy/run away"), leading to some more sensible ones ("offer him another toy instead"). In *Step 3*, each solution is evaluated for its pros and cons ("if you hit him he'll cry and not want you back in his house again"). In *Step 4*, the best option is chosen and carried out. Finally, for *Step 5*, the solution is reviewed for its effectiveness and amended as necessary.

• *Handling common tricky situations.* There are several recurring situations where children's behaviour may be especially difficult for a family, *e.g.* mealtimes, out in public, dawdling, difficulties going to bed and waking at night, lying and stealing, sibling rivalry, etc. Handling these can be practised in advance with a range of the strategies described above.

• *Wider principles of parenting.* Several more strategic aspects beyond moment-to-moment interaction are covered. These include supervision and how this changes with age (*e.g.* For how long should a 3-year-old be out of view—no more than two minutes? How do parents set up their activities to enable this level of monitoring? Should an 8-year-old be allowed to play with another child for half an hour on the way home from school?); planning joint activities; reducing sibling rivalry; promoting friendships with other children; and how to deal with school and teachers.

COMMONLY ENCOUNTERED REASONS FOR POOR PROGRESS, AND SOME SOLUTIONS

(a) Able to interact well in the clinic, but not at home. Under the stressful conditions obtaining at home, some parents are too overwhelmed by other demands to be able to practise the new skills at home. *Solutions:* (i) Start off with small, manageable tasks, which encourage parents by showing they can succeed. (ii) Problem-solve reducing other stresses (apply for nursery place for small children, get their own mother to help out, etc.). (iii) Prioritize which difficulty to focus on and ignore the rest for the time being, *e.g.* the single most important thing may be management of the child's night-waking so the mother can herself get some sleep and stop being exhausted all the time. (iv) Get a friend or neighbour along to the sessions, so s/he can support the parents in practising the new techniques back at home. (v) Do a few home visits and help parents gain confidence using the methods *in vivo.*

(b) Specific problem with one particular child, but not the others—for example, where the mother dislikes the child so much that she cannot bring herself to do things differently. *Solutions:* Several avenues may need to be explored, including: (i) Helping the mother to see the occasions when the child is behaving well may be facilitated by keeping a diary. (ii) Helping her to see that all the child's behaviour is not within the child's control, *e.g.* where appropriate by explaining that it is the hyperactivity that makes her/him behave that way. (iii) Through role-play, getting her to experience what it is like to be treated in such a rejecting way. (iv) Exploring whether the child may be the scapegoat for bad feelings originating elsewhere and about which s/he can do nothing, *e.g.* a son is felt to be just like his evil father.

(c) Has responsive parenting skills, but unable to set limits. This may be related to the parent's own upbringing or beliefs. Thus, some single mothers with only children are emotionally overinvolved, and cannot bear the thought of upsetting the child by being firm, for example by sending them to their own bedroom at night; or parents who were harshly brought up themselves cannot bring themselves to impose clear discipline, equating it with painful punishment; or parents who are unsure of themselves cannot hold back from angry responses to child taunts, thus reinforcing the power of the child. *Solution:* Talk through the parent's feelings with them. Usually they are only too aware of the issue and want to examine it, which helps them think how they might do it differently in future.

(d) General lack of parenting skills, but other relationships reasonable. Such adults may be inexperienced at the parenting role, for example if it is their first child, or they have recently adopted children, or they never looked after children when they were growing up themselves. *Solutions:* Repeated practice in as wide a range of situations as possible. Support from other, more experienced parents.

(e) Interparental inconsistency. One parent has one set of rules, which are promptly undermined by the other. *Solution:* Both parents must be seen together and helped to agree a compromise.

(f) Difficulties in all relationships. Some of the hardest to help parents are simply blind to their children's needs and behaviour, and have difficulty understanding other adults and themselves. Even when replayed scenes on video, they have difficulty spotting both friendly overtures and antisocial moves made by the child (Wahler and Sansbury 1990). Typically they are isolated, without friends, and seldom have satisfactory or enduring intimate relationships. Recent research shows that often such people were brought up in an insensitive, dismissive way by their own parents (van Ijzendoorn 1995). *Solution:* It is hard to improve the situation with short-term behavioural treatment—longer-term psychological therapy may be needed.

(g) Difficulties both in relationships and in organizing daily living. Such parents may be leading too chaotic and disorganized a lifestyle to be able to bring about consistency and shape to any aspect of their life, be it finances, care of the house fabric, or parenting. *Solution.* Usually these cases are very hard to shift. Goals for change have to be modest (but specific), and serious consideration must be made of whether it is in the child's best interests to remain in the family.

WAYS OF DELIVERING INTERVENTION
Format and duration
The above programme can be delivered as group or individual work.

• *Group work.* For moderately severe difficulties a group approach working with parents alone can be effective. The programme used in our clinic comprises a two-hour session once a week over 12 weeks for the parents of around six to eight children. Videotapes are shown of parents handling their children the 'right' and 'wrong' way, then parents are invited to role-play these in the group and practice them at home (Webster-Stratton 1984). The advantages of the group approach are cost-effectiveness and the support that parents give each other. The disadvantages are that parents are not seen directly with their children, and there is little opportunity to explore deeper personal issues.

• *Individual work.* For severe difficulties an individualized approach where the parent/s and child are seen together allows one to go at the pace of the parent/s, observe precisely how they are relating to their child, and modify the intervention accordingly. This can be especially helpful where the child responds differently from the majority, *e.g.* if s/he is hyperactive, has a hearing or learning disability, or has autistic traits. An individualized approach also enables one to do more work on other issues impinging on parenting such as interparental consistency, sibling relationships, coming to terms with abuse in the parent's own childhood, etc.

The duration of intervention can vary considerably. My own experience with individual work would fit that of Patterson *et al.* (1982) who found a median of 21 hours of treatment were necessary to achieve substantial improvements (carefully defined using observational methods). In our clinic, we use a video suite with a one-way mirror. The parents are given a small earphone, through which they receive suggestions on how to handle their child 'live' while they are looking after her/him.

• *Other types of intervention.* More intensive interventions are available. Day-patient facilities may have parents and children in for one or more days a week for about three months. Inpatient or residential units (mostly run by social services) may admit whole families for work over three to six months.

Engaging the parents

Sitting with parents telling them what to do is largely ineffective. They may agree with your suggestions in the clinic, but fail to put them into practice at home. As a doctor it is easy to slip into 'I'm the expert in charge here' mode. This can be very effective when dealing with severe physical illness, but is often counterproductive with parenting difficulties as it can make parents feel sensitive about their abilities.

One should try to be as accessible to parents as possible—a visit to the family in their own home before beginning treatment may save a lot of time later. It is worth attempting to establish a collaborative relationship (Herbert 1995), which is not unlike that between a PhD supervisor and a student: the professional contributes general expertise, but the parent is recognized as knowing their specific child best and being in charge of the upbringing. The aims of the intervention are explicitly shared with parents, so both sides are working together towards a common goal. It is helpful if possible to offer sessions to fit in with their daily routine and offer a child-minding service for their other children. Travelling expenses should be refunded if necessary. If they fail to attend, it is worth phoning them up the next day to discover what the difficulty is and how it might be overcome.

During sessions, as well as covering specific aspects of the immediate interaction between parent and child as described above, the clinician should also continually be addressing the parents' reactions to the material and exploring their beliefs and feelings about bringing up their child (Webster-Stratton and Herbert 1994). This combination of specific techniques and emotional support is essential, since trials show that straight behavioural or instructional programmes on their own have limited impact due to low compliance by parents (Wells and Egan 1988). Equally, offering only general counselling and support to parents produces little change (Dadds and McHugh 1992, McCord 1992). Both elements are necessary.

Who should provide treatment?

Conduct disorder is common, and where there are no complicating factors such as hyper-activity or emotional problems, and the aetiology is social, then arguably the Health Service should not become involved as it has limited resources. Parenting programmes for mild to moderate difficulties are available in the voluntary sector. A review by Smith and Pugh (1996) identified 50 voluntary organizations in the UK offering group parenting programmes. The approaches used varied widely from behavioural to counselling, directive to non-directive, and fixed sessions to *ad hoc* contact. Few have been satisfactorily evaluated. The responsibility for organizing assessments and interventions for serious parenting difficulties lies with social services departments. However, a referral is often made to Child and Adolescent Mental Health Services (CAMHSs) where the disturbance of child behaviour is severe or complicated by other psychiatric difficulties. Many of the effective theories and interventions around parenting have originated from health disciplines such as psychology and psychiatry, and some CAMHSs offer specialized parenting programmes. With the drive towards prevention, there is increasing interest in less specialized services providing parenting support, for example Health Visitors.

Results of parent training programmes for conduct problems
There is a wide diversity of parenting programmes, with different aims and methods. Those for child behaviour problems have been the most thoroughly evaluated. In the USA, good improvements in the quality of parenting have consistently been found in behaviourally based parent-training programmes, with effect-sizes of 0.5–0.8 of a standard deviation on measures that include questionnaires, semi-structured interviews and direct observation (Webster-Stratton *et al.* 1989, Patterson *et al.* 1993, Kazdin 1995). Child behaviour problems have improved markedly, with around half of subjects being restored to the normal range of functioning. In the UK, our own experience suggests that good gains are made in child behaviour after parent-training programmes similar to the kind described here, with good maintenance of effectiveness at one year follow-up but some decline three years later.

Other treatments for conduct disorder
PARENT- AND FAMILY-BASED
Family counselling and social work
This is often very helpful to address the grosser disruptive influences. It can then provide a setting for more specific therapeutic work.

Family therapy
This is frequently used but has hardly been evaluated. Judging from clinical experience, it is often useful in fairly well-functioning families where after only a few sessions parents may collaborate in setting clear boundaries for their child and improve the emotional atmosphere; it is less useful for chaotic, disorganized families who lack coping skills. Some varieties of family therapy depend on the parents being able to think about the difficulties and reflect on them in a new way, which many of the families find difficult. Often more concrete and practical therapies which offer parents ways of doing things differently are better accepted (Chamberlain and Rosicky 1995).

CHILD-BASED
Behaviour modification
This refers to taking one or two specific antisocial behaviours, and setting up a regime to alter them (Douglas 1989). While it can be very effective for a handful of difficulties, it does not address the wider aspects of parenting, nor the emotional issues for either the parents or the child. Consequently, it does not usually generalize to change the range of behaviours that constitute conduct disorder.

Problem-solving skills training and social skills training
Both of these forms of training have been shown to have definite although so far modest

effects (Webster-Stratton and Hammond 1997). They are only suitable for older children (say at least 8–10 years old), and are best used in conjunction with some form of family work or parent training (Kazdin *et al.* 1992).

Individual psychotherapy
Individual psychotherapy is usually unfruitful as these children have little insight into why they behave the way they do. Furthermore, when they can identify what is upsetting them, they are not usually in a position to modify it or find another way of coping. This is not to say that listening to the child and making her/him feel understood is not beneficial, but to have any major impact the child's concerns need to be fed back to the family who then need to change things accordingly.

Medication and diet
A number of drugs have been tried for aggressiveness and conduct problems but none has been shown to be at all effective in a properly conducted trial. Tranquillizers and sedatives simply do what their names suggest and also often lose their effectiveness over a few weeks as tolerance develops. They have no part to play in the management of conduct disorder. Deplorably, some children who have both conduct disorder and severe learning disability (mental handicap) are still sometimes given these drugs, often in an institutional setting. Very occasionally in adolescents who have very rapid mood swings with aggressive disinhibition, lithium (usually used for mania) has been tried, but its use for this indication remains controversial and is rare.

When children are hyperactive as well as conduct disordered, it may be appropriate to treat their restlessness and inattention with medication or diet (see Chapter 2). When stimulant medication reduces restlessness and inattention, it may well reduce defiance, aggression and antisocial behaviour too. There is no evidence that stimulants reduce conduct problems in children who are not also hyperactive. When diet helps hyperactivity, it often also reduces irritability.

SCHOOL-BASED PROGRAMMES
Behaviour in school is a major predictor of adult outcome, and children who are persistently disruptive in class have a poor outcome (Loeber and Dishion 1983). Yet the same child may show up to four times more aggression with one teacher than with another, on the same day (Werthamer-Larsson *et al.* 1991). This is due to the teachers having different levels of skill in handling the pupils, and consequently different levels of respect from them.

There are methods to help teachers manage classrooms that have been proven effective (Durlak 1995). Some have a behavioural slant, while others concentrate on getting the teachers and pupils to communicate with each other better and then set mutually agreed standards of behaviour and solutions if children are difficult in class (Gray *et al.* 1994). Sadly, many teachers are not equipped with these skills by their training. With the increasing emphasis on integration of children with special needs into manistream schools, their dissemination will become a matter of urgency.

Some schools have designated teachers with responsibility for special education, in the

UK known as Special Educational Needs Coordinators (SENCOs), who have these skills; educational psychologists also may have them, but they are often too busy conducting full assessments of special educational needs to be able to train teachers.

Occasionally, health professionals may be able to offer advice to the school, and this can be powerful in improving behaviour. Basic skills such as ignoring some irritating but minor behaviours, and praising the child while s/he is getting on with her/his work, can have significant effects (Hall *et al.* 1968).

Where there are coexistent learning difficulties, these need to be remedied through specific extra teaching. Otherwise, the child will continue not to understand most of what goes on in class, with the short-term consequence that her/his behaviour is likely to remain disruptive because s/he is bored and unoccupied, the medium-term consequence that her/his self-esteem will be low, and the long-term consequence that s/he will leave school with few or no qualifications and so be likely to be unemployed and possibly turn to crime (Granat and Granat 1978, Spreen 1988, Hinshaw 1992, Sylva and Hurry 1995).

Community-based programmes

There are beginning to be community-based preventive programmes with several elements, but these are yet to be evaluated. Preschool education programmes for disadvantaged children (such as the High Scope/Perry preschool project—Schweinhart and Weikart 1993) can have significant effects on teenage antisocial behaviour and adult criminality (Sylva 1994).

Prognosis and outcome

CONTINUITY

Looking forwards, 40 per cent of children with conduct disorder become recidivist delinquent young adults who have ongoing behaviour problems and disrupted relationships. Looking backwards, the continuity is much higher, so that 90 per cent of delinquent young adults had conduct disorder as children (Robins 1978, 1991; Loeber 1991).

TYPES OF ADULT OUTCOME

Homotypic continuity is seen more in boys (*i.e.* the symptoms remain much the same). It is characterized by aggressiveness and violence, often with an antisocial personality; alcohol and drug abuse are common, as are repeated criminal acts.

Heterotypic continuity is seen more in girls (*i.e.* different types of symptoms come to predominate). It is characterized by a wide range of emotional and personality disorders, but with less aggressiveness and criminality than in boys.

In addition to being at greater psychiatric and forensic risk, individuals with a history of conduct disorder are also more likely to be socially impaired in adulthood, being more likely to have few if any educational qualifications, a poor job history, and impaired social relations, *e.g.* more marital breakup.

PREDICTORS OF OUTCOME

In the child

A poor outcome is predicted by early onset, a wide range and high total number of symptoms, greater severity and frequency of individual symptoms, pervasiveness across situations (home, school and other), and associated hyperactivity. Conversely, having only one area of problem behaviour, such as aggressiveness alone, has a good prognosis provided there are no problems in other areas, including peer relationships and educational achievements. The presence or absence of a constellation of problems is what is important.

In the family
A poor outcome is predicted by parental psychiatric disorder, parental criminality, high hostility, and high discord directed to the child.

Conclusion
Rigorous evaluation using randomized controlled trials has shown that behaviourally based parenting programmes considerably improve both the quality of parenting experienced and the behaviour and outcome for the child. Effective programmes address both the moment-to-moment minutiae of parents' handling of children, and the wider context of their lives which can get in the way of good parenting. The task now is to disseminate effective interventions and convince purchasers of their cost-effectiveness and human value.

FURTHER READING

Herbert, M. (1987) *Conduct Disorders of Childhood and Adolescence: a Social Learning Perspective. 2nd Edn.* Chichester: Wiley
Kazdin, A.E. (1995) *Conduct Disorders in Childhood and Adolescence, 2nd Edn.* London: Sage.

REFERENCES

Achenbach, T.M. (1991) *Manual for the Child Behaviour Checklist 4–18.* Burlington, VT: University Associates in Psychiatry.
American Psychiatric Association (1994) *Diagnostic and Statistical Manual of Mental Disorders—DSM IV.* Washington, DC: American Psychiatric Association.
Azar, S., Rohrbeck, C. (1986) 'Child abuse and unrealistic expectations: further validation of the parent opinion questionnaire.' *Journal of Consulting and Clinical Psychology,* **54**, 867–868.
Barkley, R. (1997) *Defiant Children A Clinician's Manual for Assessment and Parent Training.* New York: Guilford Press.
Berenbaum, H. (1996) 'Childhood abuse, alexithymia, and personality disorder.' *Journal of Psychosomatic Research,* **41**, 588–595.
Bohman, M. (1996) 'Predisposition to criminality: Swedish adoption studies in retrospect.' *In:* Bock, G.R., Goode, J.A. (Eds.) *Genetics of Criminal and Antisocial Behaviour. Ciba Foundation Symposium 194.* Chichester: John Wiley, pp. 99–114.
Chamberlain, P., Rosicky, J. (1995) 'The effectiveness of family therapy in the treatment of adolescents with conduct disorders and delinquency.' *Journal of Marital and Family Therapy,* **4**, 441–459.
Cicchetti, D., Howes, P.W. (1991) 'Developmental psychopathology in the context of the family: illustrations from the study of child maltreatment.' *Canadian Journal of Behavioural Science,* **23**, 257–281.
—— Lynch, M. (1993) 'Toward an ecological/transactional model of community violence and child maltreatment.' *Psychiatry,* **56**, 96–118.
Crittenden, P.M. (1988) 'Relationships at risk.' *In:* Belsky, J., Nezworski, T. (Eds.) *Clinical Implications of Attachment Theory.* Hillsdale, NJ: Erlbaum, pp. 136–174.
—— Claussen, A.H., Sugarman, D.B. (1994) 'Physical and psychological maltreatment in middle childhood and adolescence.' *Development and Psychopathology,* **6**, 145–164.

Dadds, M.R., McHugh, T.A. (1992) 'Social support and treatment outcome in behavioral family therapy for child conduct problems.' *Journal of Consulting and Clinical Psychology*, **60**, 252–259.

DiLalla, L.F., Gottesman, I.I. (1989) 'Heterogeneity of causes for delinquency and criminality: lifespan perspectives.' *Developmental Psychopathology*, **1**, 339–349.

Dinwiddie, S., Bucholz, K. (1993) 'Psychiatric diagnoses of self-reported child abusers.' *Child Abuse and Neglect*, **17**, 465–476.

Dishion, J., Patterson, G.R., Grieser, P.C. (1994) 'Peer adaptation in the development of antisocial behavior: a confluence model.' *In:* Huesmann, L.R. (Ed.) *Aggressive Behavior: Current Perspectives.* New York: Plenum Press, pp. 61–95.

Dodge, K.A., Lochman, J.E. (1994) 'Social–cognitive processes of severely violent, moderately aggressive and non-aggressive boys.' *Journal of Consulting and Clinical Psychology*, **62**, 366–374.

Douglas, J. (1989) *Behaviour Problems in Young Children.* London: Routledge.

Dowdney, L., Skuse, D. (1993) 'Parenting provided by adults with mental retardation.' *Journal of Child Psychology and Psychiatry*, **34**, 25–47.

Durlak, J. (1995) *School-based Prevention Programs for Children and Adolescents.* Thousand Oaks, CA: Sage Publications.

Farrington, D.P. (1994) 'Early developmental prevention of juvenile delinquency.' *Criminal Behaviour and Mental Health*, **4**, 209–227.

Forehand, R.L., McMahon, R.J. (1981) *Helping the Noncompliant Child. A Clinician's Guide to Parent Training.* London: Guilford Press.

Gardner, F.M.E. (1987) 'Positive interaction between mothers and conduct-problem children: Is there training for harmony as well as fighting?' *Journal of Abnormal Child Psychology*, **15**, 283–293.

Gardner, H., Forehand, R., Roberts, M. (1976) 'Time-out with children: effects of an explanation and brief parent training on child and parent behaviors.' *Journal of Abnormal Child Psychology*, **15**, 283–293.

Gelles, R. (1992) 'Poverty and violence toward children.' *American Behavioral Scientist*, **35**, 258–274.

Goodman, R. (1997) 'The Strengths and Difficulties Questionnaire: a research note.' *Journal of Child Psychology and Psychiatry*, **38**, 581–586.

—— Scott, S. (1997) *Child Psychiatry.* Oxford: Blackwell Scientific.

—— —— (1998) 'Comparing the Strengths and Difficulties Questionnaire and the Child Behavior Checklist: is small beautiful?' *Journal of Abnormal Child Psychology. (In press.)*

Goyette, C.H., Conners, C.K., Ulrich, R.F. (1978) 'Normative data on revised Conners Parent and Teacher Rating Scales.' *Journal of Abnormal Child Psychology*, **6**, 221–236.

Granat, K., Granat, G.S. (1978) 'Adjustment of intellectually below-average men not identified as mentally retarded.' *Scandinavian Journal of Psychology*, **19**, 221–236.

Gray, G., Miller, A., Noakes, J. (1994) *Challenging Behaviour in Schools—Teacher Support, Practical Techniques and Policy Development.* London: Routledge.

Hall, R., Panyan, M., Rabon, D., Broden, M. (1968) 'Teacher applied contingencies and appropriate classroom behavior.' *Journal of Applied Behavior Analysis*, **1**, 315–322.

Herbert, M. (1987) *Behavioural Treatment of Children with Conduct Problems: a Practice Manual. 2nd Edn.* London: Academic Press.

—— (1995) 'A collaborative model of training for parents of children with disruptive behaviour disorders.' *British Journal of Clinical Psychology*, **34**, 325–342.

Hinshaw, S. (1992) 'Externalizing behaviour problems and academic underachievement in childhood and adolescence: causal relationships and underlying mechanisms.' *Psychological Bulletin*, **111**, 127–155.

Hobbs, S., Forehand, R., Murray, R.G. (1978) 'Effects of various durations of time-out on the non-compliant behavior of children.' *Behavior Therapy*, **9**, 652–656.

Kazdin, A. (1995) *Childhood Disorders in Childhood and Adolescence.* Thousand Oaks, CA: SAGE Publications.

—— (1997) 'Psychosocial treatments for conduct disorder in children.' *Journal of Child Psychology and Psychiatry*, **38**, 161–178.

—— Siegel, T., Bass, D. (1992) 'Cognitive problem-solving skills training and parent management training in the treatment of antisocial behavior in children.' *Journal of Consulting and Clinical Psychology*, **60**, 733–747.

Loeber, R. (1991) 'Antisocial behavior: more enduring than changeable?' *Journal of the American Academy of Child and Adolescent Psychiatry*, **30**, 393–397.

—— Dishion, T. (1983) 'Early predictors of male adolescent delinquency: a review.' *Psychological Bulletin*, **94**, 68–99.

Lyons-Ruth, K. (1996) 'Attachment relationships among children with aggressive behavior problems: the role of disorganized early attachment patterns.' *Journal of Consulting and Clinical Psychology*, **64**, 64–73.

Mandel, H. (1997) *Conduct Disorder and Under-achievement: Risk Factors, Assessment, Treatment and Prevention*. New York: John Wiley.

McCord, J. (1992) 'The Cambridge–Somerville study: a pioneering longitudinal experimental study of delinquency prevention.' *In:* McCord, J., Tremblay, R.E. (Eds.) *Preventing Antisocial Behaviour—Interventions from Birth through Adolescence*. New York: Guilford Press, pp. 196–206.

McGee, R.A., Wolfe, D.A. (1991) 'Psychological maltreatment: toward an operational definition.' *Development and Psychopathology*, **3**, 3–18.

Okun, A., Parker, J., Levendosky, A.A. (1994) 'Distinct and interactive contributions of physical abuse, socioeconomic disadvantage, and negative life events of children's social, cognitive and affective adjustment.' *Development and Psychopathology*, **6**, 77–98.

Patterson, G.R. (1982) *Coercive Family Process*. Eugene, OR: Castalia.

—— Chamberlain, P.A., Reid, J.B. (1982) 'A comparative evaluation of a parent-training program.' *Behavior Therapy*, **13**, 638–650.

—— Dishion, T.J., Chamberlain, P. (1993) 'Outcomes and methodological issues relating to treatment of antisocial children.' *In:* Giles, T.R. (Ed.) *Handbook of Effective Psychotherapy*. New York: Plenum, pp. 43–88.

Petersen, L., Gannoni, A.F. (1992) *Manual for Social Skills Training in Young People: Stop Think Do*. Camberwell, Victoria, Australia: ACER.

Reid, J.B., Kavanaugh, K., Baldwin, D.W. (1987) 'Abusive parents' perceptions of child problem behaviors: an example of parental bias.' *Journal of Abnormal Child Psychology*, **15**, 457–466.

Richman, N., Stevenson, J., Graham, P. (1982) *Pre-school to School: a Behavioural Study*. London: Academic Press.

Robins, L.N. (1978) 'Sturdy childhood predictors of adult antisocial behavior: replications from longitudinal studies.' *Psychological Medicine*, **8**, 611–622.

—— (1991) 'Conduct disorder.' *Journal of Child Psychology and Psychiatry*, **32**, 193–212.

Routh, C., Hill, J., Steele, H., Elliott, C.E., Dewey, M.E. (1995) 'Maternal attachment status, psychosocial stressors and problem behaviour: follow-up after parent training courses for conduct disorder.' *Journal of Child Psychology and Psychiatry*, **36**, 1179–1198.

Rutter, M., Cox, A., Tupling, M., Berger, M., Yule, W. (1975) 'Attainment and adjustment in two geographical areas.' *British Journal of Psychiatry*, **126**, 493–509.

—— Quinton, D. (1984) 'Parental psychiatric disorder: effects on children.' *Psychological Medicine*, **14**, 853–880.

—— Yule, W. (1975) 'The concept of specific reading retardation.' *Journal of Child Psychology and Psychiatry*, **16**, 181–197.

—— Maughan, B., Mortimer, P., Ouston, J., Smith, A. (1979) *Fifteen Thousand Hours: Secondary Schools and their Effects on Children*. Cambridge, MA: Harvard University Press.

Scarboro, M., Forehand, R. (1975) 'Effects of response-contingent isolation and ignoring on compliance and oppositional behavior of children.' *Journal of Experimental Child Psychology*, **19**, 252–264.

Scheinhart, L.J., Weikart, D.P. (1993) *A Summary of Significant Benefits: the High Scope/Perry Pre-school Study through Age 27*. Ypsilanti, MI: High Scope.

Scott, S. (1994) 'Mental retardation.' *In:* Rutter, M., Taylor, E., Hersov, L. (Eds.) *Child and Adolescent Psychiatry: Modern Approaches. 3rd Edn.* Oxford: Blackwell Scientific, pp. 616–646.

Smith, C., Pugh, G. (1996) *Learning to Be a Parent: a Survey of Group-based Parenting Programmes*. London: National Children's Bureau.

Spieker, S., Booth, C. (1988) 'Maternal antecedents of attachment quality.' *In:* Belsky, J., Nezworski, T. (Eds.) *Clinical Implications of Attachment Theory*. Hillsdale, NJ: Erlbaum, pp. 93–135.

Spreen, O. (1988) 'Prognosis of learning disability.' *Journal of Consulting and Clinical Psychology*, **56**, 836–842.

Sylva, K. (1994) 'School influences on children's development.' *Journal of Child Psychology and Psychiatry*, **35**, 135–170.

—— Hurry, J. (1995) *Early Intervention in Children with Reading Difficulties*. London: School Curriculum and Assessment Authority.

Thomas, A., Chess, S., Birch, H.G. (1968) *Temperament and Behavior Disorders in Childhood*. New York: New York University Press.

van Ijzendoorn, M.H. (1995) 'Adult attachment representations, parental responsiveness, and infant attachment: A meta-analysis on the predictive validity of the adult attachment interview.' *Psychological Bulletin*, **117**, 387–403.

Wahler, R. (1980) 'The insular mother: her problems in parent–child treatment.' *Journal of Applied Behaviour Analysis*, **13**, 13–22.

—— Sansbury, L.E. (1990) 'The monitoring skills of troubled mothers: their problems in defining child deviance.' *Journal of Abnormal Child Psychology*, **18**, 577–589.

Walker, E., Downey, G., Berman, A. (1989) 'The effects of parental psychopathology and maltreatment on child behavior: a test of the diathesis–stress model.' *Child Development*, **60**, 15–24.

Webster-Stratton, C. (1984) 'Randomized trial of two parent-training programs for families with conduct-disordered children.' *Journal of Consulting and Clinical Psychology*, **52**, 666–678.

—— Hammond, M. (1997) 'Treating children with early-onset conduct problems: a comparison of child and parent training interventions.' *Journal of Consulting and Clinical Psychology*, **65**, 93–109.

—— Herbert, M. (1994) *Troubled Families—Problem Children. Working with Parents: a Collaborative Process.* Chichester: John Wiley.

—— Hollinsworth, T., Kolpacoff, M. (1989) 'The long-term effectiveness and clinical significance of three cost-effective training programs for families with conduct-problem children.' *Journal of Consulting and Clinical Psychology*, **57**, 550–553.

Wells, K., Egan, J. (1988) 'Social learning and systems family therapy for childhood oppositional disorder: comparative treatment outcome.' *Comprehensive Psychiatry*, **29**, 138–146.

Werthamer-Larsson, L., Kellam, S.G., Wheeler, L. (1991) 'Effect of classroom environment on shy behavior, aggressive behavior, and concentration problems.' *American Journal of Community Psychology*, **19**, 585–602.

White, G., Nielsen, G., Johnson, S.M. (1972) 'Timeout duration and the suppression of deviant behavior in children.' *Journal of Applied Behavior Analysis*, **5**, 111–120.

World Health Organization (1993) *The ICD-10 Classification of Mental and Behavioural Disorders.* Geneva: WHO.

Zeanah, C.H., Zeanah, P.D. (1989) 'Intergenerational transmission of maltreatment.' *Psychiatry*, **52**, 177–196.

2
ATTENTION DEFICIT–HYPERACTIVITY DISORDER

Jody Warner-Rogers

"Pay attention!" "Please stay seated during dinner." "Look both ways before crossing the street."

The ability to regulate behaviour in accordance with the changing demands and constraints of their environment is a crucial skill for children to master. One way in which parents, teachers and other caregivers encourage the development of behavioural control is by providing a safe, structured environment in which various methods, such as the three instructions above, are used to help children identify what behaviours are appropriate, when and where. Expectations for behavioural control vary across age, settings and cultures. Seven-year-old children are unlikely to control their behaviour independently in every setting. However, 7-year-olds should demonstrate more control over their actions than 4-year-olds, albeit less than 12-year-olds. Yet, approximately 17 per cent of school-age children will exhibit a combination of poor attentional skills, overactivity and/or impulsiveness, and for these children developing the ability to independently control and modulate their behaviour will present a serious challenge (Taylor *et al.* 1991).

'Hyperactivity' is word often applied to this triad of symptoms, and the term has come to denote an enduring tendency to behave in an overactive, inattentive, restless and impulsive manner (Schachar 1991, Taylor 1994). Most children exhibit a degree of hyperactivity in some situations, and epidemiological studies indicate that this tendency is continuously distributed in the population (*e.g.* Taylor *et al.* 1991). Much of what is thought of as 'hyperactivity' may be due to inherited, biological predispositions towards this style of behaving (Sherman *et al.* 1997). The confusion arises when one attempts to distinguish categorically levels of hyperactivity within the normal range of child behaviour from levels which lie at the extremes of or even outside this range. For children with significant, pervasive hyperactivity, learning to modify their behaviour in response to environmental demands presents a serious developmental challenge that can have long-term implications for their behavioural, emotional and educational adjustment (Barkley *et al.* 1990).

Despite clear evidence that childhood hyperactivity is a serious developmental risk factor, controversy exists regarding the most appropriate manner in which to evaluate and treat these difficulties. The purpose of this chapter is to review the behavioural strategies applicable for the evaluation and management of children with hyperactivity and other attentional disorders. First, terms and diagnoses used in this area are covered, followed by a brief outline of the epidemiology of childhood hyperactivity. The discussion then moves to the clinical assessment of attention and hyperactivity. Assessment techniques that are relevant for initial evaluation, as well as those appropriate for ongoing monitoring of behavioural change are presented. Behavioural treatment strategies are then reviewed in detail. The chapter concludes with a case example that illustrates how different therapies may be combined in the comprehensive treatment of childhood hyperactivity.

Terms and concepts

HYPERACTIVITY, ATTENTION DEFICIT–HYPERACTIVITY DISORDER AND HYPERKINETIC DISORDER

The first published scientific account of children with inattentiveness, overactivity and lowered inhibition appeared over 90 years ago (Still 1902). A clinical syndrome characterized by the presence of childhood hyperactivity appeared 30 years ago in the second edition of the American Psychiatric Association's *Diagnostic and Statistical Manual* (DSM-II; APA 1968). The fourth, and current edition of the DSM (APA 1994) includes the category 'Attention Deficit–Hyperactivity Disorder' (ADHD) to apply to children whose high frequency of inattentive behaviours and/or levels of impulsivity/hyperactivity are viewed as being: (a) pervasive, (b) developmentally inappropriate, (c) functionally impairing, and (d) early in onset. Three subtypes of ADHD are included in the DSM-IV to reflect the prominence of symptom presentation. If attentional problems without concomitant hyperactivity are evident, then the 'primarily inattentive' subtype applies. If impulsivity and overactivity are dominant, then 'primarily hyperactive/impulsive' subtype can be used. The presence of all three core symptoms is captured by the 'mixed hyperactive/inattentive' subtype.

In European countries, the most widely used diagnostic classification scheme is that given in the 10th edition of the *International Classification of Diseases* (ICD-10; WHO 1988). Within the ICD scheme, the category Hyperkinetic Disorder (HK) is used to diagnose children who exhibit pervasive difficulties in all three of the core areas, inattention, impulsivity and overactivity. The criteria for HK are more inclusive, and therefore more stringent, than the general criteria for ADHD. The ADHD mixed hyperactive/inattentive subtype would be the most similar diagnostically to HK.

Despite originating from the North American diagnostic nomenclature, the term ADHD has entered the lexicon of professionals and parents in the UK. Thus it is imperative that those involved in the assessment and management of children with behavioural difficulties appreciate the subtle, but important distinctions between the terms *hyperactivity*, which refers to a tendency to behave in an overactive, inattentive and impulsive manner, *ADHD*, which should be considered in cases where some features of hyperactivity are pervasive, developmentally inappropriate, of early onset and functionally impairing, and *HK*, which is similar to ADHD, but more inclusive. [Those interested in a more detailed review of the history behind the conceptualization and diagnosis of ADHD symptoms are referred to Barkley (1990a) and Sandberg and Barton (1996).] Throughout this chapter the terms hyperactivity and ADHD will be used interchangeably, but will always refer to elevated levels of inattentive, impulsive and/or hyperactive behaviours that are both pervasive and impairing.

Clinical diagnoses of both ADHD and HK are based on overt, behavioural symptomatology. Specific psychological, neurological, neuroimaging, neurochemical or physiological investigations can inform diagnostic decisions by helping to rule out alternative explanations for hyperactive behaviour. However, at this time, the diagnosis of ADHD or HK cannot be made based solely on the outcome of such investigations. Discussion of the three core symptoms of ADHD helps to clarify the relationship between overt behavioural manifestations of hyperactivity and the underlying cognitive processes that may or may not underpin behaviour.

ATTENTION

Attention is a multidimensional construct used to describe a wide variety of both cognitive and behavioural phenomena. Several different aspects and types of attention have been identified, including: general level of arousal; ability to engage and disengage one's attention (*i.e.* focused attention); ability to maintain attention over time (*i.e.* sustained attention); ability to attend to one relevant stimulus in the presence of competing, but irrelevant stimuli (*i.e.* selective attention); and attentional capacity (*i.e.* working memory). An important distinction must be made between inattentive behaviours and the cognitively based attentional processes that are assumed to underpin these behaviours. The term inattentive behaviour encompasses a wide range of behaviours, including: lack of persistence in activities such as play or school work; orientation to task-irrelevant stimuli; engagement in task-irrelevant activity; and frequent change of activities (Taylor 1994).

Empirical efforts to establish which, if any, aspect of attention is actually deficient in children with hyperactivity have generated mixed results. Performance on psychological tests of attention can be very context-specific, and subtle environmental variations, such as whether an adult is present during assessment or whether the task is structured or un- structured, can greatly affect performance. Initially, sustained attention—that is, the ability to maintain attention over time—was considered to be impaired in children with hyperactivity (Douglas and Peters 1979). Deficits in the ability to control and direct attention have also been implicated (Loge *et al.* 1990). Others (*e.g.* Sergeant and Scholten 1985) have argued that hyperactive children fail to allocate enough attention to tasks, either at the beginning or during a task.

Yet, research has demonstrated that children with ADHD can concentrate as well as non-ADHD children if the task or activity to which they are supposed to be directing their attention is highly salient and stimulating, such as a television programme (Landau *et al.* 1992). Moreover, those children who do evidence deficits on specific cognitive tests of attention are more likely to have global impairments in their cognitive functioning rather than specific weaknesses in attentional processing skills (*e.g.* Halperin *et al.* 1990). Such conflicting results led to the consideration that cognitive processes outside the realm of attention may actually underlie inattentive behaviour. Contemporary theories purport that impulsiveness, rather than inattentiveness, may be the primary area of difficulty in hyperactive children (*e.g.* Barkley 1997a).

IMPULSIVITY

The behaviour of hyperactive children is characterized by poorly regulated responses. Such children seem to have difficulty withholding inappropriate responses, and appear to 'behave without thinking'. The term 'impulsiveness' is often applied to such a style of behaviour.

Here again, a distinction must be made between the cognitive processes involved in behavioural control and the overt manifestations of poorly controlled behaviour (*e.g.* difficulty waiting turn, jumping in prematurely).

Barkley (1997a) has argued that poorly regulated behaviour is underpinned by core deficits in three cognitive processes involved in behavioural inhibition. First, children with ADHD have difficulty inhibiting a prepotent response, or a response that is likely to bring immediate reinforcement. Second, these children have difficulty stopping an ongoing response, even when provided with feedback that the responses are no longer appropriate. Due to this difficulty, they do not permit themselves a delay in which to consider the tasks at hand and plan or implement new, more appropriate responses. Third, children with ADHD have difficulty with interference control; that is, when they actually do stop ongoing responses— thus permitting themselves that important delay in which they could consider the task at hand—they seem unable to use the delay period very effectively because it is so easily disrupted by competing responses or events (*i.e.* 'interference').

An alternative, more behavioural conceptualization of impulsivity suggests that hyperactive children have a preference for immediate reward and are motivated by a need to keep experiences of delay at a minimum (Sonuga-Barke *et al.* 1996). This does not imply a cognitive deficit in impulse control (Sonuga-Barke 1996), rather it highlights the functionality of impulsive behaviours and underscores critical individual differences in preferences and willingness to tolerate delay. This is an area of intense debate and research, the results of which will have potentially important implications for assessment and treatment of hyperactivity.

OVERACTIVITY

Overactivity refers to an excess of movements, either in minor, task-irrelevant movements (*e.g.* toe-tapping, fidgeting) or in gross body movements (*e.g.* restlessness) (Taylor 1994). This observation of increased motor movements is not a result of rater bias. Objective, mechanical measurement of children rated by others as hyperactive demonstrates that these children do make more movements than non-hyperactive children (*e.g.* Taylor *et al.* 1991). This increase in movements cannot be a secondary function of poorly controlled attention, as it is observed both during the day (*e.g.* Taylor *et al.* 1991), and during sleep (*e.g.* Porrino *et al.* 1983) when there are no demands on attention or behavioural control.

Epidemiology

PREVALENCE

Figures regarding the prevalence of childhood hyperactivity vary widely depending on the definitions used and the populations sampled. For example, estimates of hyperactivity in clinic-referred children differ in critical ways from estimates describing rates in community-based samples. The factors that influence which children get referred for services (*e.g.* presence of comorbid emotional difficulties, poor parental coping, significant peer problems at school) must also be taken into account (Woodward *et al.* 1997). The number of children who exhibit a high level of hyperactive behaviours is greater than the number of children who would actually meet diagnostic criteria for ADHD and HK.

31

Data from a large epidemiological, community-based study conducted in London indicate that approximately 17 per cent of 7-year-old male children exhibit pervasive hyper-activity (Taylor *et al.* 1991). In comparison, around 3–9 per cent of children exhibit ADHD (Szatmari *et al.* 1989) and only 1.7 per cent meet diagnostic criteria for HK (Taylor *et al.* 1991). Estimates indicate that the ratio of affected boys to girls is 4:1 (Ross and Ross 1982, James and Taylor 1990).

AGE OF ONSET

The age at which hyperactivity first manifests can vary. A DSM-IV diagnosis of ADHD requires that pervasive hyperactive behaviours be present by the age of 7 years (APA 1994), implying that the onset of difficulties is in early childhood. ADHD symptoms have been identified by parents when children are as young as 4 years (Sullivan *et al.* 1990). Over-activity and inattention are commonly identified concerns by parents and teachers in preschool children, but for most children, such issues are less of a problem by the time they reach 5 years of age. (For a review of behavioural problems in preschoolers, see Campbell 1995.)

ASSOCIATED DIFFICULTIES

Hyperactivity is associated with a wide variety of other childhood difficulties. The initial assessment of a hyperactive child must therefore be systematic and comprehensive, so that comorbid difficulties can be identified and alternative diagnoses ruled out (Weinberg and Emslie 1991). Some problems may coexist with ADHD (*e.g.* oppositional behaviour, reading difficulties), while others have diagnostic priority over ADHD. For example, the DSM-IV stipulates that a diagnosis of ADHD should not be made if the hyperactivity symptoms occur in the context of a pervasive developmental disorder, like autism. This is not to say that children with pervasive developmental disorders do not exhibit ADHD-like symptoms that warrant intervention. Rather, the diagnostic distinction serves to establish a hierarchy of difficulties which in turn has important implications for treatment.

The most common difficulties presenting comorbidly with ADHD are oppositionality and noncompliance. Collectively, studies suggest that 40–90 per cent of children with ADHD meet diagnostic criteria for oppositional defiant disorder or conduct disorder (for a review, see Tannock 1998). Such behavioural difficulties often persist into adolescence, with estimates indicating that 68 per cent of adolescents with ADHD have a comorbid oppositional defiant disorder (Barkley *et al.* 1991). Often it is difficult to distinguish acts of volitional noncompliance from the more thoughtless rule-breaking characteristic of impulsivity. Children with ADHD often fail to comply with requests because they simply forget the entire instruction or have difficulty inhibiting a response. Children may present with a combination of both types of noncompliance. Longitudinal research suggests that ADHD is a risk factor for the development of conduct disorder (Loeber *et al.* 1994). These findings highlight the need to identify early indications of conduct problems, such as aggression, and target these areas in treatment.

Academic difficulties are also associated with ADHD (Cantwell and Baker 1991). Over one-third of clinically-referred children diagnosed with ADHD have comorbid reading difficulties (August and Garfinkel 1990). Behaving in an inattentive and impulsive manner may contribute to poor performance in the classroom. However, specific learning disabilities coexist with hyperactivity. If such specific learning difficulties are not identified early in the assessment process, then any treatment that focuses on decreasing hyperactive behaviours in the classroom will not necessarily result in concomitant improvements in academic attainment.

Difficulties in making and/or keeping friends are also generally noted in children with ADHD. Peer problems may be particularly evident when ADHD presents in combination with specific learning disabilities (*e.g.* Flick 1992) or aggression. Children with ADHD tend to be more argumentative, dominating, aggressive and disruptive, which can lead to social rejection and isolation (Guevremont 1990). Their impulsiveness may affect their ability to process socially relevant cues and information accurately, and lead to tendencies to view neutral or ambiguous social interactions in a negative or hostile manner (Milich and Dodge 1984).

OUTCOME

The developmental outcome of ADHD in childhood can vary widely. Though an estimated 30 per cent of children with a diagnosis of ADHD will have outgrown their difficulties by adolescence (Barkley *et al.* 1990), a substantial proportion continue to experience problems with attention and behavioural control as they develop. Adolescents with a history of ADHD are at risk for the development of behavioural and mood difficulties (Biederman *et al.* 1996), and are more likely than non-hyperactive teenagers in the community to engage in antisocial acts (*e.g.* theft, vandalism) and substance abuse (Barkley *et al.* 1991). Some of the earlier studies failed to differentiate the effects of pure ADHD from those better accounted for by comorbid conduct problems. However, a recent longitudinal epidemiological study found that hyperactivity is itself a risk factor for later developmental problems, independent of the presence of conduct disorder (Taylor *et al.* 1996).

ADHD in adulthood is now beginning to receive more research, clinical and media attention (Denckla 1991, Hallowell and Ratey 1994). Early estimates indicate that around 3 per cent of adults may be affected, though inattention, distractibility and impulsivity are likely to be more prominent than motoric overactivity (Feifel 1996). However, the general adjustment of some individuals who manifest ADHD symptoms in adulthood, but who emerged from adolescence without other comorbid difficulties (*e.g.* conduct problems, learning difficulties), may be unaffected. With the demands of formal education behind them, such individuals might settle into an occupational niche which appropriately and positively accommodates their style of impulsive decision making, need for stimulation and high energy level. Forthcoming findings from ongoing investigations should shortly provide more insight into these issues.

Assessment

Given the heterogeneity of problems characteristic of and associated with childhood hyperactivity, a thorough assessment necessitates a multidisciplinary, multimodal and multi-informant approach. Goodman and Scott (1997) suggest that a comprehensive assessment focuses on five key areas: (1) symptoms ("What sort of problem is it?"); (2) impact ("How much distress or impairment does it cause?"); (3) risks ("What factors have initiated and maintained the problem?"); (4) strengths ("What assets are there to work with?"); (5) explanatory model ("What beliefs and expectations do the family bring with them?"). The specific techniques used to answer such questions may vary depending on the nature of the referral and the professionals involved, but can include: parental interview, parental rating scales, school report, teacher rating scales, teacher interview, interview with the child, physical examination of the child and formal psychometric evaluation. With the exceptions of cognitive testing, which is the professional responsibility of a clinical or educational psychologist, and the physical examination, which is in the domain of a medical professional, the other techniques can be used by professionals from a wide range of disciplines. A brief overview of a variety of assessment techniques is presented below. Barkley (1990a) offers a more comprehensive review.

The results of an initial assessment will help to guide diagnostic decisions regarding the presence of ADHD or HK by establishing whether or not hyperactive behaviours are present with sufficient severity and pervasiveness, are developmentally impairing, and are not better accounted for by other disorders (e.g. pervasive developmental disorder). Treatment planning follows directly from the formulation. Interventions must be individualized, based on the child's unique profile of strengths and weaknesses, and should take into consideration the views, values and resources of the child and family. Ongoing assessment throughout treatment is necessary to monitor behavioural change.

CLINICAL INTERVIEW

Information regarding hyperactive behaviours can come from many sources, but the views of parents and teachers are particularly important. The structure of clinical interviews can vary. There is no specific diagnostic interview for ADHD. However, general guidelines for assessing ADHD symptomatology via interviews are available (see Barkley 1990a). There is a method of standardized interviewing, the Parental Account of Childhood Symptoms (PACS, Taylor et al. 1986) which, with appropriate training in administration and inter-pretation, can provide reliable information on a child's hyperactive behaviour in the home.

With regard to parental interviews, one general strategy is to commence with basic demographic data, then move to the primary referral concerns of the parents (Barkley 1988). Questions about the specific behaviours that are leading parents and/or others to indicate that the child is 'hyperactive' should focus on the descriptions of these behaviours, the situations in which they occur, and their consequences. In particular, it may be helpful to ask parents about specific situations in which hyperactive behaviours are likely to occur, such as playing (alone or with others), mealtimes, getting dressed, bathing, when parent is on the telephone, when family is visiting others, at bedtime, or at any other time in which demands on behavioural control are high. Asking parents to describe their child's behaviour and their subsequent attempts to manage it provides an opportunity to examine potentially problematic parent–child interactions, especially if rates of noncompliance are high and parental discipline ineffective. This information can then be used in the development of a functional analysis of factors which may be eliciting or maintaining current behavioural patterns.

The crux of the parental interview is the gathering of a detailed developmental history and information on the level of impairment caused by the hyperactivity. The child's progress in many different areas of development (*e.g.* motor, language, social, emotional) must be addressed. Medical histories obtained from a child's GP can serve to corroborate parental reports of any developmental delay. Details of the events prompting the referral can highlight issues in family circumstances, parental ability to cope, and the chronicity of behavioural difficulties.

The opinions and views of teachers and other professionals within the school setting should always be solicited. Teachers can be asked to provide written reports, but it is often useful to clarify their input by speaking with them directly. Information on how the child behaves in structured situations where demands on attention are high (*e.g.* maths lessons), as well as less structured situations where demands on attention might be low (*e.g.* free play), is also useful. In particular, asking teachers to provide specific examples of a child's behaviour in a variety of activities, such as quiet group work, quiet work on a task set by the teacher, quiet work on a task that the child chooses, and group work on tasks that are set and chosen by the child, can be helpful (Taylor *et al.* 1991). Teacher impressions of a child's academic progress and social interactions are imperative in establishing the pervasiveness of difficulties.

The child may also be interviewed directly, depending on age. One must take into account that children and adolescents tend not to be the most reliable reporters of the frequency or intensity of their own behavioural problems (Barkley *et al.* 1991). Nonetheless, their views regarding school, interactions with friends and relationships within the family are extremely important. They may feel frustrated that, although they complete their homework, they get into trouble because they have lost the assignment before they get the chance to turn it in. They may want more friends, but not appreciate how their impulsive, boisterous behaviour pushes others away. They may feel that everyone is always angry with them because they are 'naughty'. Such subjective senses of failure, isolation and unfairness can easily damage the child's self-image and may go overlooked if the child's views are not actively sought.

RATING SCALES AND QUESTIONNAIRES
There are several different rating scales available to assess general behavioural problems as well as the specific symptoms of hyperactivity and ADHD. The utility of rating scales lies in one's ability to ascertain whether the frequency or intensity of a child's behavioural difficulties, as seen by the person rating them, vary significantly from the range of normal child behaviour. Using the normative data provided for rating scales, a comparison is made between a particular child's score and the scores obtained by a group of same-age (but not always same-gender) children. One then determines whether the particular child's score is statistically deviant from this group of scores. Although many of these rating scales have been standardized on American children, they are used widely within Great Britain. Rating scales are useful in screening for behavioural difficulties, and the data provided can greatly supplement information gathered during interviews and direct observation. Diagnostic decisions, however, should never be made based only on a score or set of scores from rating scales.

In terms of general behaviour screening questionnaires and rating scales, the Rutter scales (Rutter *et al.* 1970), available in both parent (A2) and teacher (B2) forms, are widely used in a variety of settings (Elander and Rutter 1996). The Strengths and Difficulties Questionnaire (SDQ) is a relatively new instrument that taps behavioural, emotional and social functioning and measures positive, as well as negative, characteristics (Goodman 1997). The SDQ is quick to administer (about 25 minutes), and teacher and parent forms are available for children between the ages of 4 and 16. There is also a self-report form that can be administered to children between the ages of 11 and 16. Both the Rutter scales and the SDQ have been standardized on British children. The Behavior Problems scale of the Achenbach Child Behavior Checklist (CBCL) is a longer and more detailed instrument (118 items), which can be useful for screening for general psychopathology (Achenbach and Edlebrock 1983), and computerized scoring programmes are available.

Amongst questionnaires specifically designed to assess hyperactivity symptoms, the revised Conners rating scales (Conners 1997), originally developed to assess outcome in medication trials (Conners 1969), are very widely used. Quick to administer, they can be used repeatedly to monitor behavioural change and treatment progress. Several different versions are available, but it is the 48-item version for which the best normative data are published (Goyette *et al.* 1978). Parallel parent and teacher forms are available. The Home Situations Questionnaire (HSQ) and School Situations Questionnaire (SSQ), developed by Barkley (1997b), are also useful in that they draw particular attention to the settings (*e.g.* mealtimes, homework time, travelling in the car) in which problems may occur.

CAVEATS ABOUT RATING SCALES AND QUESTIONNAIRES

It is not uncommon for two sources (*e.g.* parents and teachers) to provide disparate behavioural ratings for the same child. This can occur for several reasons. First, the child may be behaving quite differently in different situations. If this is the case, more systematic investigation of the environmental factors that may be functioning to elicit or reinforce particular behavioural patterns in each setting will be indicated. Second, different expectations may operate in different settings. For example, if the child has four tantrums a week, a parent might describe tantrums as occurring 'sometimes', whereas a teacher may describe the same frequency as 'very often'. Third, research indicates that individuals from different cultural backgrounds may respond differently to the rating scales (Sonuga-Barke *et al.* 1993). Rating scales are also subject to halo effects, with the presence of noncompliance or other oppositional behaviour operating to inflate ratings of hyperactivity (Abikoff *et al.* 1993). Irrespective of the cause, if the responses from different sources are very disparate, then direct observation of behaviour in each situation may be the best manner in which to determine what is going on.

PSYCHOLOGICAL TESTING

General cognitive assessment serves to quantify a child's level of intellectual functioning. This is important because the diagnosis of ADHD requires that the child's inattentive, impulsive and overactive behaviours be out of keeping with their developmental level. In addition, an appreciation of a child's actual level of cognitive functioning has implications for establishing appropriate expectations for behaviour and for planning treatment. One of the most widely used tests for assessing general intellectual functioning is the Wechsler Intelligence Scale for Children, Third Edition (WISC-III; Wechsler 1992). This also provides a 'Freedom from Distractibility' factor score; however, although the name suggests a link between distractibility and hyperactivity symptoms, in fact low scores on this factor can occur for a wide variety of reasons and should not be interpreted as a specific cognitive marker for ADHD (Kaufman 1994).

Given the association between ADHD and specific learning disorders (Szatmari *et al.* 1989, Taylor *et al.* 1991), it is important that a child's level of academic attainment, particularly in the areas of reading and spelling, be considered. One can make predictions about the level of academic functioning expected based on both a child's chronological age and 'mental age' (*i.e.* general intellectual abilities). These predictions can be compared to actual academic abilities as assessed by academic attainment tests, such as the Wechsler Objective Reading Dimensions (WORD) test (Wechsler 1996). Discrepancies between expected ability and actual attainment serve as indicators for the presence of specific learning difficulties, which must also be addressed in the treatment plan.

In addition to general psychometric testing, specialized neuropsychological assessment of attentional processes and response inhibition can provide useful data regarding a child's particular profile of cognitive strengths and deficits. However, as stated previously, the diagnosis of ADHD or HK is based on *behavioural* manifestations, and the link between overt behaviour and underlying cognitive processes, albeit heavily researched, is still theoretical. As noted earlier, one must also remember that factors other than impaired attention or inhibition, such as low motivation, oppositionality, or anxiety, can affect test performance. Although many neuropsychological tests are sensitive to ADHD symptoms, they are not necessarily specific to such symptoms (*e.g.* Matier-Sharma *et al.* 1995), and assessments of problem behaviours in the naturalistic setting (*e.g.* home, school) may provide more ecologically valid measures (Barkley 1991).

A few commonly employed neuropsychological assessments are briefly reviewed in Appendix 2.1 (p. 53).

BEHAVIOURAL OBSERVATION
Direct observation of a child's behaviour can provide a unique opportunity to identify associations between aspects of the immediate environment and the occurrence of behavioural difficulties. Factors and situations that seem to elicit particular problem behaviours can be considered. For example, off-task behaviours in the classroom may appear to be triggered by a child's apparent inability to cope with the task set. Aggressive interactions with peers may be elicited because the child has not waited for his/her turn in a game and disrupted the group activities. Furthermore, observation of the consequences that immediately follow a child's behaviour can lead to the development of hypotheses regarding the factors that may be maintaining problematic behaviours or limiting appropriate behaviours. For example, a child engaging in off-task behaviour may attract the attention of other pupils in the class and make them laugh. Such inappropriate behaviour may be one of the few ways the child is able to gain attention from his/her peers. This attention may function as a positive

reinforcer and increase the likelihood that the child will again engage in such inappropriate behaviours. It is also possible that prosocial behaviours may not be acknowledged or reinforced sufficiently, thus decreasing the likelihood that such behaviours will increase.

There are some formal coding schemes available for quantifying the direct observation of hyperactivity symptoms (for a review, see Barkley 1988). Although typically such structured coding schemes are not required for the general assessment of hyperactivity, they can be very useful for research purposes, when a more exact measurement of interpersonal interactions is indicated. For the purpose of clinical assessment of hyperactivity in younger children, direct observation of play skills can be quite informative. Children with hyperactivity may have difficulty sticking to one theme for any length of time and may instead change activities rapidly or explore play areas in a quick, disorganized manner. Direct observation of parent–child interactions is a component of the parent training interventions outlined below and can be incorporated into child management strategies used in the classroom.

FROM ASSESSMENT RESULTS TO TREATMENT PLANS
The heterogeneity of difficulties characteristic of childhood hyperactivity necessitates that treatment plans be individually tailored to meet each child's particular needs. The results from a multidisciplinary assessment can lead directly to the development of a comprehensive treatment plan. The overall goal of any intervention for hyperactivity is symptom reduction. No therapy is an actual 'cure' for the disorder. Optimizing a child's development by systematically expanding their repertoire of appropriate behaviours and enhancing the family's ability to cope with the hyperactivity are the focus of treatment. Information gathered during the initial assessment can serve as baseline data against which treatment progress should be compared. Ongoing monitoring of behavioural change should be an integral part of any treatment plan.

As hyperactive children often have a variety of associated difficulties, a multimodal approach to treatment will generally be indicated. The first, and potentially most important step in any treatment plan should be educating parents, teachers and the children themselves about ADHD and the child's own unique pattern of strengths and vulnerabilities. Armed with this understanding, parents and teachers are in a better position to develop realistic, attainable goals for a child's behaviour and long-term development. Professionals and caregivers must take into consideration both the need to address difficulties firmly and the desire to develop a child's areas of particular strengths. Insuring that the child is in an appropriate educational placement should also be an item for early attention in any treatment plan.

Treatment
In general, three main treatment options are available—psychological approaches, psycho-pharmacology, and nutritional interventions. Behavioural interventions are the main focus of this chapter, though nutritional and pharmacological approaches are discussed briefly. Often a combination of behavioural treatments and psychopharmacological interventions prove the most effective in decreasing ADHD symptomatology (Abramowitz *et al.* 1992). For example, a multimodal approach to treatment of ADHD might include the following

aspects: medication, remedial academic tutoring, social skills training, parenting training and counselling, a school behaviour monitoring programme, and individual work with the child to address issues of self-esteem and their understanding of ADHD (Hechtman 1993).

NUTRITIONAL INTERVENTIONS

Initially, nutritional interventions for hyperactivity were based on the assumption, put forward by Feingold (1975), that the disorder was caused by food allergies to salicylates, preservatives and artificial food colouring in the diet. The idea was intrinsically appealing, though clinical trials failed to demonstrate the efficacy of the Feingold diet (for a review, see Kado and Takagi 1996). This is not to say that there is no role for dietary therapy in the treatment of hyperactivity. Rather, one can conclude that general exclusion diets, when applied across the board, are not very effective. Highly individualized dietary manipulations may, however, help a few children. In a well-designed study of hyperactive children thought to have some sort of food allergy, Carter *et al.* (1993) found that the behaviour of some of these children (24 per cent) did improve when they were placed on a 'few foods' elimination diet and worsened when an identified target food was reintroduced into the diet.

Unfortunately, at present the empirical evidence available is insufficient to develop general guidelines for nutritional interventions. If parents express an interest in dietary manipulations, they can be encouraged to develop a food diary to investigate any association between food and behaviour. If such an association does appear to be present, then a mental health professional can assist in monitoring behaviour patterns more formally over time and a dietician can be consulted to develop a specifically tailored intervention (Taylor *et al.* 1998).

PSYCHOPHARMACOLOGY

Psychopharmacology is by far the most common treatment for ADHD in the USA (Safer and Krager 1988). In contrast, behavioural interventions, which are recommended and applied less frequently in the USA (Barkley *et al.* 1991), have been the treatment of choice in the UK. This disparate use of behavioural therapies across the two cultures reflects differences in diagnostic conceptualization and problem formulation. Historically, the European view of the more general difficulties associated with ADHD has been focused on the difficulties associated with educational and conduct problems (Prendergast *et al.* 1988), whereas medication was reserved for those children meeting the more stringent criteria for HK. This view may now be changing, at least within the medical community. Professionals with expertise in this area agree that psychopharmacological intervention is helpful for some children with ADHD even if these children do not meet the more stringent criteria for HK (Sayal and Taylor 1997).

The main pharmacological intervention for childhood hyperactivity is stimulant medications, of which methylphenidate (Ritalin) is the most commonly prescribed. Estimates suggest that approximately 88 per cent of those children diagnosed with ADHD by a primary care physician in the USA are prescribed methylphenidate (Wolraich *et al.* 1990). A substantial research base documents the effectiveness of methylphenidate in improving the core symptoms characteristic of hyperactivity, as well as in ameliorating some of the associated cognitive and social interaction problems (for a review, see Schachar *et al.*

39

1996). Stimulant medication has also been shown to decrease disruptive behaviour and increase time spent on task (Pelham *et al.* 1985), and can improve the academic productivity of some children with ADHD (Pelham *et al.* 1985, Evans and Pelham 1991) and enhance their attention during play activities (Pelham *et al.* 1990).

Aside from methylphenidate, another stimulant medication used occasionally is dextro-amphetamine. Other psychopharmacological interventions include the tricyclic antidepressants, desipramine and imipramine, and clonidine (Elia 1991, Taylor *et al.* 1998). Such medications, though acknowledged to be appropriate choices for treatment, have not been studied as intensively as methylphenidate.

One of the major disadvantages of stimulant medication is that the treatment effects are short-lived, and typically disappear as soon as the medication wears off. Furthermore, although stimulant medications are effective in reducing the behavioural symptoms, there is no indication that children use these periods of enhanced behavioural control to acquire new self-control skills (Schachar *et al.* 1996). Some stimulant medications can also exacerbate or contribute to the onset of tics. Thus, for a variety of reasons, environmental interventions are often indicated to facilitate more long-lasting behavioural change. Behaviourally based psychological therapies can be implemented on their own, or easily and effectively combined with stimulant medication (Abramowitz *et al.* 1992, Carlson *et al.* 1992).

BEHAVIOURAL APPROACHES

Behavioural interventions have proved successful in many clinical outcome studies, though direct comparison across studies is often difficult because of the complexity and variation characteristic of such interventions (Whalen and Henker 1991). Target behaviours selected for treatment, the implementors of treatments (*e.g.* teacher, parent, therapist), the setting in which treatment occurs (*e.g.* classroom, home), treatment techniques, the duration of treatment and the frequency of sessions can all vary widely (Schachar *et al.* 1996). The heterogeneity of ADHD and sampling techniques (*i.e.* whether studies use clinic or community based samples) can confound issues further and make generalization difficult (Whalen and Henker 1991, Woodward *et al.* 1997). Nonetheless, the interventions discussed here can be viewed as useful components of a multimodal treatment approach, in which different skills and behaviours can be targeted and a variety of techniques incorporated simultaneously.

The assumptions, objectives and general approaches underpinning environmental interventions for ADHD have been succinctly summarized by Horn *et al.* (1991): if the skills required to regulate behaviour are deficient in children with ADHD, then such skills must be directly taught or shaped. From a social learning perspective, teaching the child specific self-regulation skills, such as those believed to be lacking in ADHD, is often targeted by training parents and teachers to reward appropriate behaviour and punish inappropriate behaviour. These types of treatments are geared towards improving behaviour somewhat indirectly, because they actually target the behaviour of those dealing with the child and the features of the child's immediate environment.

In contrast, a cognitive-behavioural approach focuses more directly on the child by teaching self-control and problem-solving skills (Horn *et al.* 1991). Areas that can be targeted include impulsivity and self-control (*i.e.* anger management, use of nonaggressive problem-solving techniques), for which a self-instructional approach can be applied (Kendall and Braswell 1985, Braswell and Bloomquist 1991); self-esteem, for which a cognitive–behavioural approach can be used; and peer relationships, for which social skills training may be indicated (Guevremont 1990). The development of adaptive skills is another area that may benefit from intervention, as children with ADHD and normal intellectual abilities have been found to exhibit deficits in their ability to carry out tasks involved in daily living (Roisen *et al.* 1994, Stein *et al.* 1995).

Parent education
Parenting a hyperactive child can be an extremely stressful endeavour (Fischer 1990), and consideration of the social–family context is a key feature of clinical assessment. In addition, parents may have their own problems above and beyond those directly associated with their hyperactive child (*e.g.* alcoholism, depression). If parental distress or dysfunction is of sufficient severity, a separate referral to adult mental health services may be warranted, as the professionals involved in the care of the child might not be in the best position to address specific and individual needs of adult family members. Furthermore, these difficulties would most likely require treatment before the parent could effectively engage in and adhere to behaviourally oriented interventions involving their child.

In general, when educating parents about ADHD, information about the symptoms, aetiology, clinical course, prognosis and treatment options should be provided (Taylor *et al.* 1998). Several excellent books written specifically for parents of children with ADHD are available (*e.g.* Douglas 1991, Barkley 1995, Taylor 1997). These resources can be extremely useful supplements to, but never a replacement for, open and ongoing dialogue between professionals and caregivers. Many parents appreciate the opportunity to meet others in similar situations, and local ADHD parent support groups have been started in several areas. A substantial amount of information on ADHD and hyperactivity can now be found on the internet. It may be prudent to warn parents in advance that these various sources of information may sometimes offer confusing or conflicting advice regarding the disorder and the different management options. When questions arise, parents should always be encouraged to discuss them with the professionals involved in their child's care.

Parent training in child management
A large component of helping parents cope with the symptoms of hyperactivity involves encouraging them to use the most effective techniques for managing those behaviours that are most problematic. The basic strategies for parenting a child with hyperactivity include: (a) providing a high degree of positive attention and consequences to compliance and other desirable behaviours; (b) developing clear, concise and consistent expectations for behaviour; and (c) utilizing nonphysical negative consequences for problem behaviours in a nonpunitive fashion (Taylor *et al.* 1998). Teaching parents to use these strategies is one of the hallmarks of behavioural parent training, an intervention that has proven to be an extremely effective treatment for school-age children with ADHD in reducing both parent-reported behavioural problems and parenting stress (Anastopoulos *et al.* 1993). Several books are available that were written specifically for parental, as opposed to professional, audiences (*e.g.* Barkley

1997b, Taylor 1997). The techniques outlined in such parent-oriented manuals are prescriptive in nature. Although some families will be able to implement the strategies and suggestions independently, the majority will benefit from the opportunity to receive individual help from a skilled clinician, who can modify and tailor the techniques to meet the specific needs of the child and abilities of the parents.

General features of parenting skills programmes
The actual teaching of these specific child management techniques can take many forms (for a review on parent training, see Callias 1994). Three well-known parent training manuals have been widely used by professionals for working with parents and their children with ADHD (Forehand and McMahon 1981, Patterson 1982, Barkley 1997b). The parent training programmes outlined in these manuals are geared towards children between the ages of 3 and 11 who exhibit oppositional, noncompliant behaviour but do not have significant emotional problems. Modifications can be made to the programmes when working with older children such that the child's role in programme development and negotiation of consequences is enhanced (Robin and Foster 1989).

The general steps in teaching effective child management skills to the parents of ADHD children include the following: (1) specific problem situations must be identified and the behaviours that occur within these situations described and measured; (2) the consequences, both positive and negative, for behaviour in these situations must be identified; (3) the parent–child relationship must be considered; (4) parents should be taught practical and effective ways of communicating their expectations for child behaviour, reinforcing appropriate behaviours and reducing undesirable ones. In many families, there will be an imbalance between low levels of positive consequences following appropriate, desirable behaviours and a relatively high frequency and/or intensity of negative consequences following inappropriate or problematic behaviours. One goal of treatment will be to reverse this ratio, and increase the degree of positive attention and consequences following appropriate behaviour. Taylor *et al.* (1998) emphasize that if positive interactions between a parent and child are infrequent, then parents may need input to develop their ability to attend positively to their child's behaviour. Specific playtime exercises, designed to help parents identify and reinforce their child's positive behaviour, can be used to help them attend to and encourage appropriate child behaviour. Parents can then focus on developing, practising and consistently implementing specific child management techniques, such as giving one command at a time, token systems, response cost and time out.

Of the available parent training resources, the most widely *empirically validated* is the 10-step programme designed by Barkley (1990a, 1995). Research indicates that it can result in improvements in ADHD symptomatology, increases in parental self-esteem and competence, and decreases in parental stress (Anastopoulos *et al.* 1993). The exact mechanisms by which these results are attained are not clear, though one hypothesis is that the acquisition of effective parenting skills allows parents to manage behavioural difficulties more efficiently, and subsequently they view their child's behaviour as less severe (Anastopoulos *et al.* 1993). The general structure and highlights of the Barkley programme are summarized here, although it must be stressed that this outline review should in no way be construed as a replacement for the excellent practical manuals that are available (Barkley 1990a, 1997b), which include assessment devices, monitoring forms, parental handouts and homework tasks.

Briefly, the 10-step parent training approach (Anastopoulos and Barkley 1990, Barkley 1997b) starts with an initial session that provides an overview of the programme and helps to educate parents about ADHD. The second session is devoted to helping the parents understand how deviant child behaviour develops and is maintained and introduces the principles of behaviour management, including behaviour monitoring. The third step focuses on developing the parents' ability to attend to positive behaviours and ignore negative behaviours within the framework of a child's playtime exercise. The fourth step involves extending the skills acquired in the third session to free play situations and teaching parents to give commands in a clear, simple and direct manner. At the fifth step, parents learn to establish a 'token economy' system in the home.

Token economies are schemes in which targeted behaviours are reinforced with points, stickers or actual tokens. These things may not have any intrinsically rewarding function, but they can be relatively easily earned and accumulated, then 'cashed in' for 'real' rewards. Such schemes are very useful in working with hyperactive children because they combine immediacy of reward with minimal disruption. Furthermore, there can be a wider range of activities (*e.g.* special time with a parent) or tangible rewards from which to choose when cashing in tokens, thus reducing the risk that children will get bored with the scheme.

Of particular importance for working with ADHD, and critical to any parent training programme, is the feature that positive strategies for child management must be in place before the focus shifts to punishment. Thus, it is not until the sixth session of the Barkley approach that parents learn how to incorporate a response cost element into the home token economy. In the seventh step, time-out procedures for use in the home are introduced. The eighth session extends this lesson by teaching parents to use time out in public places. The ninth session is used for discussion of future behavioural problems, or other related issues (*e.g.* functioning in school). The tenth session is used for a booster meeting, and generalization of new skills across settings (from clinic, to home, to public places) is addressed.

Although skills are introduced and practised in the clinic, parents are expected to implement the techniques at home. Ongoing monitoring of child behaviour and parental use of skills in the home is often required. Thus, parent training programmes require fairly intensive parental involvement and commitment. In some cases, additional problems such as severe parental psychopathology or a high degree of parental discord may impede or compete with a parent's ability to benefit from the programme. As noted earlier, these issues are generally identified at the assessment stage and should be addressed before behavioral training is commenced.

Educational modifications
As highlighted earlier, information about a child's educational setting and academic functioning is critical to treatment planning. An important part of the assessment is determining a child's level of academic ability and current classroom performance to ensure that educational provision is appropriate. Once this has been established, the behaviour and

academic performance of children with ADHD can be targeted with a combination of minor environmental manipulations, more intensive classroom-based contingency management techniques, and, when necessary, remedial or specialized teaching to address specific learning difficulties.

Minor modifications to the structure of the classroom and the format and timing of lessons may be helpful. For example, a hyperactive child might have his/her desk placed near the front of the class. This makes it easier for the teacher to monitor the progress of work and reward on-task, appropriate behaviour. For children who are extremely distractible, being placed in a classroom with fewer pupils may help, although placing the child in a distraction-free area, completely separate from his/her peers is unlikely to be effective. Hyperactive children seem to have a preference for bright, highly stimulating materials (Zentall 1986). This preference can be incorporated into educational materials in the classroom. Some hyperactive children may also perform better in the morning and be more active in the afternoon (Porrino *et al.* 1983, Zager and Bower 1983). Where possible, altering schedules to have the more intensive academic subjects scheduled earlier in the day may be beneficial. Finally, presentation of new material in small chunks interspersed with brief breaks puts less of a strain on vulnerable concentration skills and is preferable to having longer teaching sessions.

Moment-to-moment management of a child's behaviour in the classroom may be more problematic. Consultation with teachers regarding specific behavioural management techniques is often necessary. Many of the child management strategies reviewed in the parent training section above can be modified for teachers working with hyperactive children. Specific techniques, such as contingent praise, ignoring, verbal reprimands, token economies and response cost, can all be integrated into the classroom. In terms of the empirical validation of such techniques, many of the studies investigating the effectiveness of classroom management strategies are conducted in specially-designed classrooms (*e.g.* Carlson *et al.* 1992). The consistent and effective use of such techniques can place a high demand on teachers. Hence, given the pressures involved in managing the typically large numbers of pupils in mainstream classes, some teachers may be unable to adhere to a programme that requires intensive input to one pupil. Many of the techniques are more realistic for use in special educational settings where class sizes are smaller so that the teacher is in a better position to provide immediate feedback and reinforcement to the child (Abramowitz *et al.* 1992), or in situations where a classroom aide is available.

There are several very useful reviews and guidebooks for teachers and those focusing on managing hyperactivity within the school setting (*e.g.* Gordon and Asher 1994). Developing open lines of communication between home, school and professionals should be a priority. Linking reward programmes between home and school (*e.g.* child earns points at school that can be redeemed for extra privileges at home) can also be beneficial.

Summary of behaviour management guidelines
Several basic guidelines for behaviour management of children with ADHD apply regardless of whether one is working with parents in the home or teachers in the classroom. The following top five 'rules of thumb' provide a useful summary. (1) Rules and expectations for behaviour should be clear, concise and conspicuous. In the classroom a card with a few

basic rules (*e.g.* raise your hand to ask a question, stay in your seat during lessons, etc.) can be taped to a child's desk. At home, a few critical house rules can posted on the refrigerator (*e.g.* sit down to eat your food). When possible, it is helpful to phrase rules in a positive way, emphasizing what is expected in terms of behaviour (*e.g.* "You should remain in your seat during the lesson"), rather than focus on what is not permitted (*e.g.* "You should not leave your seat during a lesson"). (2) Instructions should be kept concise. Larger tasks should be broken down into small steps. This allows more opportunities for immediate feedback (*i.e.* praise after completing each step). As new skills are acquired, the steps involved can be combined into larger chunks. (3) Consequences, both positive and negative, for behaviour need to be delivered as soon after the behaviour as possible (preferably immediately) and at a greater frequency than might be used for a non-hyperactive child. (4) Positive strategies should always be in place before punishment techniques are incorporated. (5) To help children orient to the adult speaker and to learn to appreciate the relationship between their behaviour and the responses of others around them, verbal consequences, whether positive (*i.e.* praise) or negative (*i.e.* reprimands) should be prefaced by the child's name and include reference to the behaviour in question. For example, a vague compliment like, "Well done, John, thanks" is more likely to be effective when modified to, "John, well done. I really like it when you put your toys away." The same holds true for reprimands.

Direct interventions with children
Historically, many approaches to working directly with children with ADHD have been cognitive–behavioural in nature and have emphasized self-control skills. For example, one procedure, which can be applied to the management of impulsive behaviour, is termed 'self-instruction'. This procedure involves instructing individuals in self-talk strategies to guide them through various stages of a technique for problem-solving (*e.g.* identifying a problem, and then generating, choosing, implementing and evaluating a solution). The hypothesis is that these self-talk techniques, which were practised overtly initially, would eventually become internalized and compensate for deficits in self-regulation (Hinshaw and Melnick 1992). Specific training in anger control techniques is another self-management strategy, whereby children are taught to recognize internal (*e.g.* physiological) cues of increasing anger, develop techniques for decreasing or redirecting the anger (*e.g.* walk away from situation), and rehearse these techniques in response to increasing incitement from others (Novaco 1979).

Unfortunately, although cognitive–behavioural training (CBT) has been shown in some cases to improve parental perceptions of hyperactive behaviour in the home, and has been linked to increased self-esteem in ADHD children (Fehlings *et al.* 1991), research indicates that CBT alone has little clinically significant impact on the symptoms of ADHD, particularly with regard to behaviour in the classroom (Abikoff 1991, Bloomquist *et al.* 1991). Experts (*e.g.* Hinshaw 1992) now suggest that such verbally mediated techniques, like self-talk and anger control strategies, should probably not be the initial aim in working with children, given the verbal difficulties and academic underachievement often associated with ADHD. However, this is not to say that there is no role for CBT and other child-oriented interventions in the treatment of ADHD.

The effectiveness of CBT with ADHD children may be enhanced if it is combined with other techniques, such as rehearsing new skills within and outside the clinic, having adults provide concrete reinforcement of appropriate social behaviour, and having the children self-monitor their own use of new skills (Hinshaw *et al.* 1984, Hinshaw and Melnick 1992). In addition, though clinical trials may indicate that CBT is not effective when applied in isolation, it may be very useful in individual cases and studies are currently underway to examine the efficacy of CBT as one component in a comprehensive treatment plan (Hechtman 1993). In summary, though self-regulatory processes may not always be effective in their own right, there does appear to be a role for such approaches in the multimodal management of ADHD.

The social interactions between children with ADHD and their peers can be notoriously stormy. Problems with social interaction may arise because children with ADHD have difficulties modifying their reactions in response to changes in situations or tasks (Cousins and Weiss 1993). In addition, in light of their impulsiveness, children with ADHD may not process social cues accurately and may jump to wrong conclusions regarding the intent of others, construing a hostile intent when none is actually present (Milich and Dodge 1984). Social skills training to address such issues can take place individually or in groups, and be formal or relatively informal.

Techniques to shape basic conversational skills, train social problem-solving skills and directly reinforce appropriate social behaviour may be applied (Cousins and Weiss 1993). There are some manuals available for teaching social skills (*e.g.* Jackson *et al.* 1983). Youngsters with milder ADHD may benefit from participation in supervised social activities with their peers in the community, such as scouting or hobby groups. The behaviour of children with more severe levels of hyperactivity may preclude their ability to join such groups. For these children, formal social skills programmes organized by a trained leader and developed to incorporate more structure, provide immediate feedback and reflect the particular social difficulties associated with ADHD may be more useful. Guevremont (1990) outlines one such programme, which focuses on four general skills of entering social situations, developing conversational skills, problem-solving, and conflict resolution and controlling anger. Clinical researchers are now looking at new and innovative ways to combine different behavioural treatments. In particular, efforts to combine social skills training for the child with parent training are currently being investigated (Cousins and Weiss 1993).

CASE STUDY

Ben is a 10-year-old boy with a long history of overactive, restless and impulsive behaviour who was evaluated in a hyperactivity clinic at the request of his local child mental health service. He lives at home with his mother, father and 8-year-old brother. There is no family history of psychiatric illness. A maternal uncle and first cousin had difficulties learning to read and write. Ben's mother received good prenatal care and there was no exposure to drugs or alcohol during pregnancy. His delivery was unremarkable and he reached developmental milestones in a timely manner.

Ben's mother first noted problems when he was 4 years old and began to attend nursery school. She noticed that he was not like the other children in the class. In that setting, Ben was silly, jumped around constantly and had little regard for his own safety. He was aggressive with peers and had difficulty making friends. The nursery staff noted that his attention was poor. He could concentrate for two or three minutes on some tasks, but only up to five minutes on tasks that he really enjoyed.

During the first year of primary school, he was excluded twice for aggressive behaviour. Difficulties were noted in his acquisition of basic reading skills. When he was 8 years old he was evaluated by an educational psychologist. His intellectual abilities were average, but his reading skills were two years below the levels expected given his age and general ability. A diagnosis of dyslexia was made and he began to receive three hours of support teaching a week in school.

Around the same time, his GP referred him for evaluation of his hyperactive behaviour. He was seen by a psychiatric team at a local child guidance clinic. Based on the developmental history provided by his parents, observations in the clinic, reports from school, and psychometric testing from the educational psychologist, a diagnosis of hyperkinetic disorder was made. He was started on methylphenidate (Ritalin) and responded very well. His concentration increased to 30 minutes. He was less impulsive and more appreciative of the consequences of his behaviour. His interactions with peers improved and he quickly established a circle of friends. At home, he had occasional temper tantrums and physical altercations with his younger brother. His mother was the main disciplinarian and managed these incidents by ignoring temper tantrums and sending him to his room for more major rule violations.

His progress continued to be monitored by the local child guidance clinic. At 9 years 6 months of age, his behaviour began to deteriorate. Teachers noted that his concentration was not as good as it had been. He was making self-derogatory remarks about his abilities. No specific environmental factors could be identified (*e.g.* parental discord, peer difficulties), and the dose of medication was increased. This resulted in an improvement in his concentration. He was referred for to a specialist hyperactivity clinic for a more detailed assessment of his difficulties and consultation regarding his management.

Ben and his parents were seen by a psychologist and psychiatrist at a specialist hyperactivity clinic when he was 10 years old. The appointment lasted about two and a half hours. The assessment included: parental interview; parent and teacher rating scales; a telephone interview with his teacher; psychometric evaluation of his cognitive and reading abilities; and an interview with him to discuss his understanding of hyperactivity and dyslexia and their treatment. Ben was on his usual dose of Ritalin during the assessment. His behaviour was relatively well-controlled, though reports from his parents and school indicated that off medication he became very disinhibited, impulsive, overactive and distractible. Several conclusions were made based on the results of the assessment. Recommendations were made and discussed with the family during a separate visit to the clinic.

First, Ben continued to meet the diagnostic criteria for hyperkinetic disorder. His symptoms had improved on Ritalin and it was recommended that this treatment be continued. Second, his parents had a good understanding of his disorder, but were not linked into any local support service. This option was discussed with them. The parents were doing a relatively effective job of managing his behaviour at home, but there was no formal reward scheme in place whereby he could earn privileges (*e.g.* extra computer time or play time with dad) for good behaviour. The parents felt that such a scheme would help them and others focus on Ben's appropriate behaviour and accomplishments, and they accepted an offer of several outpatient sessions designed to teach more specific child management strategies. These were arranged through the local child guidance clinic.

Third, Ben had an age-appropriate understanding of hyperkinetic disorder and its management. He did not feel stigmatized by the disorder and was always compliant with his medication. He knew another, slightly older boy with similar problems who also took medication. He thought the medication worked 'on chemicals in his brain' and helped by 'slowing him down a bit so he could think'. He gave an interesting example of how his medication helped him. He explained that his younger brother often 'wound him up'. When he was not on medication, Ben got angry easily, generally punched his brother on these occasions, and got punished. When he was on medication, he still thought about punching his brother, but typically decided not to and would simply walk away, thus avoiding punishment.

Such insight into his own decision-making processes and appreciation of the relationship between his actions and their consequences suggests that Ben may be a very good candidate for some individual, cognitive–behavioural work focusing on anger and impulse control. This work could help him to generalize the ability he shows to inhibit impulsiveness when he is on medication. Such work would also assist him to take responsibility for his own actions by highlighting the fact that although the medication helps him inhibit an impulsive reaction (*e.g.* punching his brother) and choose a more appropriate response (*e.g.* walking away), he alone is responsible for his actions, not the medication. Ben and his parents were open to this option of individual work, but felt that it would be best conducted during the summer term, when demands on family schedules were reduced. In the meantime, he was encouraged to discuss any questions he might have about hyperactivity with his parents or with professionals involved in his care. Specific interventions designed to target his social functioning were not indicated at this time. However, his self-esteem appeared vulnerable and the causes of this were explored in more depth.

Academic testing revealed that his reading abilities remained about two years behind expected levels. The school was in the process of completing a Statement of Special Educational Needs. The psychologist who evaluated Ben in the hyperactivity clinic contributed a report that supported the need for an increase in the level of specialized reading input provided to him. When talking to the psychologist, Ben revealed that he felt 'stupid' because of the dyslexia and was angry that his younger brother could read better than he could. Indeed, the self-derogatory comments Ben had made in the past seemed primarily related to his academic difficulties. Unlike hyperactivity, which he viewed as a treatable problem, he saw his dyslexia as something that could not be treated and would always be with him. The nature and management of dyslexia were discussed briefly with him at that point, but it was recommended that he have multiple opportunities to discuss his views about his strengths and weaknesses with his special needs teacher. The teachers did not express any difficulties managing his behaviour in the classroom. With a view to increasing his self-esteem in the academic setting, the need for more attention to be paid to his strengths within the school environment was highlighted in a feedback letter to the school.

Ben will continue to be monitored locally by both education and health professionals. His progress will be reviewed formally about every six months to ensure that the management plan for his combined problems of hyperactivity and reading difficulties is up-to-date. Such systematic review helps to ensure that treatment plans are modified as particular goals are met and that any new behavioural, educational or emotional needs arising in the course of development are identified and addressed.

Conclusion

Hyperactivity is a relatively common behavioural problem. For some children, however, the severity and pervasiveness of their hyperactive behaviour will present major difficulties and may warrant a clinical diagnosis of ADHD or HK. Early identification and intervention may help modify the negative risk factors associated with childhood hyperactivity. For parents, teachers and other caregivers, the treatments outlined above can help them cope with a hyperactive child by: (a) providing education about the child's unique difficulties; (b) teaching them skills for managing problematic behaviours and encouraging the development of appropriate behaviours; and (c) assisting them to develop the optimal environment for the child, both in the home and in the classroom. For hyperactive children themselves, behavioural treatments can help them behave in a more well-controlled manner in situations that place a high demand on attending, complying and withholding inappropriate responses. Comprehensive treatment plans must be individualized and are best developed when they are based upon the thorough assessment of a child's unique strengths and vulnerabilities in all domains of development, as well as a family's ability to cope with and manage that child's behaviour.

REFERENCES

Abikoff, H. (1991) 'Cognitive training in ADHD children: less to it than meets the eye.' *Journal of Learning Disabilities*, **24**, 205–209.
—— Courtney, M., Pelham, W.E., Koplewicz, H.S. (1993) 'Teachers' ratings of disruptive behaviours: the influence of halo effects.' *Journal of Abnormal Child Psychology*, **21**, 519–533.
Abramowitz, A.J., Eckstrand, D., O'Leary, S.G., Dulcan, M.K. (1992) 'ADHD children's responses to stimulant medication and two intensities of a behavioural intervention.' *Behavior Modification*, **16**, 193–203.
Achenbach, T.M., Edlebrock, E. (1983) *Manual for the Child Behavior Checklist and Revised Child Behavior Profile*. Burlington, VT: University of Vermont, Department of Psychiatry.
APA (1968) *Diagnostic and Statistical Manual of Mental Disorders, 2nd Edn*. Washington, DC: American Psychiatric Association.
—— (1994) *Diagnostic and Statistical Manual of Mental Disorders, 4th Edn*. Washington, DC: American Psychiatric Association.
Anastopoulos, A., Barkley, R.A. (1990) 'Counseling and parent training.' *In:* Barkley, R.A. (Ed.) *Attention Deficit Hyperactivity Disorder: a Handbook for Diagnosis and Treatment*. New York: Guilford Press, pp. 397–441.
—— Shelton, T.L., DuPaul, G.J., Guevremont, D.C. (1993) 'Parent training for attention-deficit hyperactivity disorder: its impact on parent functioning.' *Journal of Abnormal Child Psychology*, **21**, 581–596.
August, G.J., Garfinkel, B.D. (1990) 'Comorbidity of ADHD and reading disability among clinic-referred children.' *Journal of Abnormal Child Psychology*, **18**, 29–45.
Barkley, R.A. (1988) 'Attention deficit disorders with hyperactivity.' *In:* Mash, E.J., Terdal, L.G. (Eds.) *Behavioral Assessment of Childhood Disorders, 2nd Edn*. New York: Guilford Press, pp. 69–104.
—— (1990a) *Attention Deficit Hyperactivity Disorder: a Handbook for Diagnosis and Treatment*. New York: Guilford Press.
—— (1990b) 'A critique of current diagnostic criteria for attention deficit hyperactivity disorder: clinical and research implications.' *Journal of Developmental and Behavioral Pediatrics*, **11**, 343–352.
—— (1991) 'The ecological validity of laboratory measures and analogue assessment methods of ADHD symptoms.' *Journal of Abnormal Child Psychology*, **19**, 149–178.
—— (1995) *Taking Charge of ADHD: the Complete, Authoritative Guide for Parents*. New York: Guilford Press.
—— (1997a) 'Behavioral inhibition, sustained attention, and executive functions: constructing a unifying theory of ADHD.' *Psychological Bulletin*, **121**, 65–94.
—— (1997b) *Defiant Children: a Clinician's Manual for Assessment and Parent Training. 2nd Edn*. New York: Guilford Press.
—— Fischer, M., Edelbrock, C.S., Smallish, L. (1990) 'The adolescent outcome of hyperactive children diagnosed by research criteria. I. An 8-year prospective follow-up study.' *Journal of the American Academy of Child and Adolescent Psychiatry*, **29**, 546–557.
—— Anastopoulos, A.D, Guevremont, D.C., Fletcher, K.E. (1991) 'Adolescents with ADHD: patterns of behavioral adjustment, academic functioning, and treatment utilization.' *Journal of the American Academy of Child and Adolescent Psychiatry*, **30**, 752–761.
Biederman, J., Farone, S., Milberger, S., Curtis, S., Chen, L., Marrs, A., Ouellette, C., Moore, P., Spencer, T. (1996) 'Predictors of persistence and remission of ADHD into adolescence: results from a four-year prospective follow-up study.' *Journal of the American Academy of Child and Adolescent Psychiatry*, **35**, 343–351.
Bloomquist, M.L., August, G.J., Ostrander, R. (1991) 'Effects of a school-based cognitive–behavioral intervention for ADHD children.' *Journal of Abnormal Child Psychology*, **19**, 591–605.
Braswell, L., Bloomquist, M.L. (1991) *Cognitive Behavioral Therapy with ADHD Children*. New York: Guilford Press.
Cairns, E., Cammock, T. (1978) 'Development of a more reliable version of the Matching Familiar Figures Test.' *Developmental Psychology*, **14**, 555–560.

Callias, M. (1994) 'Parent training.' *In:* Rutter, M., Taylor, E., Hersov, L. (Eds.) *Child and Adolescent Psychiatry: Modern Approaches. 3rd Edn.* Oxford: Blackwell Scientific Publications, pp. 918–935.

Campbell, S.B. (1995) 'Behavior problems in preschool children: a review of recent research.' *Journal of Child Psychology and Psychiatry*, **36**, 113–150.

Cantwell, D.P, Baker, L. (1991) 'Association between attention deficit–hyperactivity disorder and learning disorders.' *Journal of Learning Disabilities*, **24**, 88–95.

Carlson, C.L., Pelham, W.E., Milich, R., Dixon, J. (1992) 'Single and combined effectiveness of methylphenidate and behavior therapy on the classroom performance of children with attention-deficit hyperactivity disorder.' *Journal of Abnormal Child Psychology*, **20**, 213–232.

Carter, C.M., Urbanowicz, M., Hemsley, R., Mantilla, L., Strobel, S., Graham, P.J., Taylor, E. (1993) 'Effects of a few foods diet in attention deficit disorders.' *Archives of Diseases in Childhood*, **69**, 564–568.

Conners, K. (1969) 'A teacher rating scale for use in drug studies with children.' *American Journal of Psychiatry*, **126**, 884–888.

Cousins, L.S., Weiss, G. (1993) 'Parent training and social skills training for children with attention deficit hyperactivity disorder: how can they be combined for greater effectiveness?' *Canadian Journal of Psychiatry*, **38**, 449–457.

Denckla, M.B. (1991) 'Attention deficit hyperactivity disorder—residual type.' *Journal of Child Neurology*, **6** (Suppl.), S44–S50.

Douglas, J. (1991) *Is My Child Hyperactive?* Harmondsworth: Penguin.

Douglas, V.I., Peters, K.G. (1979) 'Toward a clearer definition of the attentional deficit of hyperactive children.' *In:* Hale, E.A., Lewis, M. (Eds.) *Attention and the Development of Cognitive Skills.* New York: Plenum, pp. 173–247.

Elander, J., Rutter, M. (1996) 'Use and development of the Rutter's Parents' and Teachers' Scales.' *International Journal of Methods in Psychiatric Research*, **6**, 63–78.

Elia, J. (1991) 'Stimulants and antidepressant pharmakinetics in hyperactive children.' *Psychopharmacology Bulletin*, **27**, 411–415.

Evans, S.W., Pelham, W.E. (1991) 'Psychostimulant effects on academic and behavioral measures for ADHD junior high school students in a lecture format classroom.' *Journal of Abnormal Child Psychology*, **19**, 537–552.

Fehlings, D.L., Roberts, W., Humphries, T., Gawe, G. (1991) 'Attention deficit hyperactivity disorder: does cognitive behavioral therapy improve home behavior?' *Journal of Developmental Pediatrics*, **12**, 223–228.

Feifel, D. (1996) 'Attention deficit hyperactivity disorder in adults.' *Postgraduate Medicine*, **100**, 207–211

Feingold, B.F. (1975) 'Hyperkinesis and learning disabilities linked to artificial food flavors and colors.' *American Journal of Nursing*, **75**, 797–803.

Fischer, M. (1990) 'Parenting stress and children with attention deficit hyperactivity disorder.' *Journal of Clinical Child Psychology*, **19**, 337–346.

Flicek, M. (1992) 'Social status of boys with both academic problems and attention deficit hyperactivity disorder.' *Journal of Abnormal Child Psychology*, **20**, 353–366.

Forehand, R., McMahon, R. (1981) *Helping the Noncompliant child: a Clinician's Guide to Parent Training.* New York: Guilford Press.

Goodman, R. (1997) 'The Strengths and Difficulties Questionnaire: a research note.' *Journal of Child Psychology and Psychiatry*, **38**, 581–586.

—— Scott, S. (1997) *Child Psychiatry.* Oxford: Blackwell Scientific.

—— Stevenson, J. (1989) 'A twin study of hyperactivity. I. An examination of hyperactivity scores and categories derived from Rutter Teacher and Parent Questionnaires.' *Journal of Child Psychology and Psychiatry*, **30**, 671–689.

Gordon, S.B., Asher, M. (1994) *Meeting the ADD Challenge: a Practical Guide for Teachers.* Champaign, IL: Research Press.

Goyette, C.H., Conners, K., Ulrich, R.F. (1978) 'Normative data on revised Conners' parent and teacher rating scales.' *Journal of Abnormal Child Psychology*, **6**, 221–236.

Guevremont, D. (1990) 'Social skills and peer relationship training.' *In:* Barkley, R.A. (Ed.) *Attention Deficit Hyperactivity Disorder: a Handbook for Diagnosis and Treatment.* New York: Guilford Press, pp. 540–572.

Hallowell, E.M., Ratey, J.J. (1994) *Driven to Distraction: Recognizing and Coping with Attention Deficit Disorder from Childhood through Adulthood.* New York: Simon & Schuster.

Halperin, J.M., Newcorn, J.H., Sharma, V., Healey, J.M., Wolf, L.E., Pascualvaca, D.M., Schwartz, S. (1990) 'Inattentive and noninattentive ADHD children: do they constitute a unitary group?' *Journal of Abnormal Child Psychology*, **18**, 437–449.

Hechtman, L. (1993) 'Aims and methodological problems in multimodal treatment studies.' *Canadian Journal of Psychiatry*, **38**, 458– 464.

Hinshaw, S.P. (1992) 'Externalizing behavioral problems and academic underachievement in childhood and adolescence: causal relationships and underlying mechanisms.' *Psychological Bulletin*, **111**, 127–155.

—— Melnick, S. (1992) 'Self-management therapies and attention-deficit hyperactivity disorder: reinforced self-evaluation and anger control interventions.' *Behavior Modification*, **16**, 253–273.

—— Henker, B., Whalen, C.K. (1984) 'Self-control in hyperactive boys in anger-inducing situations: effects of cognitive–behavioural training and of methylphenidate.' *Journal of Abnormal Child Psychology*, **12**, 55–77.

Horn W.F., Ialongo, N.S., Pascoe, J.M., Greenberg, G., Packard, T., Lopez, M., Wagner, M., Puttler, L. (1991) 'Additive effects of psychostimulants, parent training and self-control therapy with ADHD children.' *Journal of the American Academy of Child and Adolescent Psychiatry*, **30**, 233–240.

Jackson, N.F., Jackson, D.A., Munroe, C. (1983) *Getting Along with Others: Teaching Social Effectiveness to Children.* Waterloo, Ontario: Research Press.

James, A., Taylor, E. (1990) 'Sex differences in the hyperkinetic syndrome of childhood.' *Journal of Child Psychology and Psychiatry*, **31**, 437–446.

Kado, S., Takagi, R. (1996) 'Biological aspects.' *In:* Sandberg, S. (Ed.) *Hyperactivity Disorders of Childhood.* Cambridge: Cambridge University Press, pp. 246–279.

Kagan, J. (1966) 'Reflection–impulsivity: the generality and dynamics of conceptual tempo.' *Journal of Abnormal Psychology*, **71**, 17–24.

Kaufman, A.S. (1994) *Intelligent Testing with the WISC-III.* New York: John Wiley.

Kendall, P.C., Braswell, L. (1985) *Cognitive–Behavioral Therapy for Impulsive Children.* New York: Guilford Press.

Landau, S., Lorch, E.P., Milich, R. (1992) 'Visual attention to and comprehension of television in attention-deficit hyperactivity disordered and normal boys.' *Child Development*, **63**, 928–937.

Loeber, R., Green, S.M., Keenan, K., Lahey, B.B. (1994) 'Which boys will fare worse? Early predictors of the onset of conduct disorder in a six-year longitudinal study.' *Journal of the American Academy of Child and Adolescent Psychiatry*, **34**, 499–509.

Loge, D.V., Staton, R.D., Beatty, W.W. (1990) 'Performance of children with ADHD on tests sensitive to frontal lobe dysfunction.' *Journal of the American Academy of Child and Adolescent Psychiatry*, **29**, 540–545.

Matier-Sharma, K., Perachia, N., Newcorn, J.H., Sharma, V., Halperin, J.M. (1995) 'Differential diagnosis of ADHD: are objective measures of attention, impulsivity and activity level helpful?' *Child Neuropsychology*, **2**, 118–127.

Milich, R., Dodge, K.A. (1984) 'Social information processing in child psychiatry populations.' *Journal of Abnormal Child Psychology*, **12**, 471–479.

Novaco, R.W. (1979) 'The cognitive regulation of anger and stress.' *In:* Kendall, P.D., Hollon, S.D. (Eds.) *Cognitive–Behavioral Interventions: Theory, Research, and Procedures.* New York: Academic Press, pp. 241–285.

Patterson, G.R. (1982) *A Social Learning Approach to Family Intervention. Vol. 3. Coercive Family Process.* Eugene, OR: Castalia.

Pelham, W.E., Bender, M.E., Caddell, J., Booth, S., Moorer, S.H. (1985) 'Methylphenidate and children with attention deficit disorder.' *Archives of General Psychiatry*, **42**, 948–952.

—— McBurnett, K., Harper, G.W., Milich, R., Murphy, D.A., Clinton, J., Thiele, C. (1990) 'Methylphenidate and baseball playing in ADHD children: who's on first?' *Journal of Consulting and Clinical Psychology*, 130–133.

Pennington, B.F. (1991) *Diagnosing Learning Disorders: a Neuropsychological Framework.* New York: Guilford Press.

Porrino, L.J., Rapoport, J.L., Behar, D., Sceery, W., Ismond, D., Bunney, W.E. (1983) 'A naturalistic assessment of the motor activity of hyperactive boys. I. Comparison with normal controls.' *Archives of General Psychiatry*, **40**, 681–687.

Prendergast, M., Taylor, E., Rapoport, J.L., Bartko, J., Donnelly, M., Zametikin, A., Ahearn, M.B., Dunn, G., Wieselberg, H.M. (1988) 'The diagnosis of childhood hyperactivity: a U.S.–U.K. cross-national study of DSM-III and ICD-9.' *Journal of Child Psychology and Psychiatry*, **29**, 298–300.

Robin, A.L., Foster, S.L. (1989) *Negotiating Parent–Adolescent Conflict.* New York: Guilford Press.

Roisen, N.J., Blondis, T.A., Irwin, M., Stein, M. (1994) 'Adaptive functioning in children with attention deficit hyperactivity disorder.' *Archives of Pediatric and Adolescent Medicine*, **148**, 1137–1142.

Ross, D.M., Ross, S.A. (1982) *Hyperactivity: Current Issues, Research and Theory*. New York: John Wiley.

Rosvold, H.E., Mirsky, A.F., Sarason, I., Bransome, E.R., Beck, L.H. (1956) 'A continuous performance test of brain damage.' *Journal of Consulting Psychology*, **20**, 343–350.

Rutter, M., Tizard, J., Whitmore, K. (1970) *Education, Health and Behaviour*. London: Longmans Green.

Safer, D.J., Krager, J.M. (1988) 'A survey of medication treatment for hyperactive–inattentive students.' *Journal of the American Medical Association*, **260**, 2256–2258.

Sandberg, S., Barton, J. (1996) 'Historical development.' *In:* Sandberg, S. (Ed.) *Hyperactivity Disorders of Childhood. Cambridge Monographs in Child and Adolescent Psychiatry.* Cambridge: Cambridge University Press, pp. 1–25.

Sayal, K., Taylor, E. (1997) 'Drug treatment in attention deficit disorder: a survey of professional consensus.' *Psychiatric Bulletin*, **21**, 398–400.

Schachar, R.J. (1991) 'Childhood hyperactivity.' *Journal of Child Psychology and Psychiatry*, **32**, 155–191.

—— Tannock, R., Cunningham, C. (1996) 'Treatment.' *In:* Sandberg, S. (Ed.) *Hyperactivity Disorders of Childhood*. Cambridge: Cambridge University Press, pp. 433–476.

Sergeant, J.A., Scholten, C.A. (1985) 'On data limitations in hyperactivity.' *Journal of Child Psychology and Psychiatry*, **26**, 111–124.

Sherman, D.K., Iacono, W.G., McGue, M.K. (1997) 'Attention-deficit hyperactivity disorder dimensions: a twin study of inattention and impulsivity–hyperactivity.' *Journal of the American Academy of Child and Adolescent Psychiatry*, **36**, 745–753.

Sonuga-Barke, E.J.S. (1996) 'When "impulsiveness is delay aversion": a reply to Schweitzer and Sulzer-Azaroff (1995).' *Journal of Child Psychology and Psychiatry*, **37**, 1023–1025.

—— Minocha, K., Taylor, E.A., Sandberg, S. (1983) 'Inter-ethnic bias in teacher ratings of childhood hyperactivity.' *British Journal of Developmental Psychology*, **11**, 187–200.

—— Williams, E., Hall, M., Saxton, T. (1996) 'Hyperactivity and delay aversion. III: The effect on cognitive style of imposing delay after errors.' *Journal of Child Psychology and Psychiatry*, **37**, 189–194.

Stein, M.A., Szumowski, E., Blondis, T.A., Roizen, N.J. (1995) 'Adaptive skills dysfunction in ADD and ADHD.' *Journal of Child Psychology and Psychiatry*, **36**, 663–670.

Still, G.F. (1902) 'The Coulstonian lectures on some abnormal psychical conditions in children.' *Lancet*, **i**, 1008–1012.

Sullivan, A., Kelso, J., Stewart, M. (1990) 'Mothers' views of the ages of onset for four childhood disorders.' *Child Psychiatry and Human Development*, **20**, 269–278.

Szatmari, P., Offord, D.R., Boyle, M.H. (1989) 'Ontario Child Health Study: prevalence of attention deficit disorder with hyperactivity.' *Journal of Child Psychology and Psychiatry*, **30**, 219–230.

Tannock, R. (1998) 'ADHD: advances in research.' *Journal of Child Psychology and Psychiatry*, **39**, 65–100.

Taylor, E.A. (Ed.) (1986) *The Overactive Child. Clinics in Developmental Medicine No. 97.* London: Mac Keith Press.

—— (1994) 'Syndromes of attention deficit and overactivity.' *In:* Rutter, M., Taylor, E., Hersov, L. (Eds.) *Child and Adolescent Psychiatry: Modern Approaches. 3rd Edn.* Oxford: Blackwell Scientific.

—— (1997) *Understanding Your Hyperactive Child: the Essential Guide for Parents. 3rd Edn.* London: Vermilion.

—— Sandberg, S., Thorley, G., Giles, S. (1991) *The Epidemiology of Childhood Hyperactivity. Maudsley Monographs, No. 33.* Oxford: University of Oxford Press.

—— Chadwick, O., Heptinstall, E., Danckaerts, M. (1996) 'Hyperactivity and conduct problems as risk factors for adolescent development.' *Journal of the American Academy of Child and Adolescent Psychiatry*, **35**, 1213–1226.

—— Sergeant, J., Doepfner, M., Gunning, B., Overmeyer, S., Mobiue, H. (1998) 'Clinical guidelines for hyperkinetic disorder.' *European Journal of Child and Adolescent Psychiatry. (In press.)*

Wechsler, D. (1992) *Manual: Wechsler Intelligence Scale for Children—3rd Edn.* Sidcup, Kent: Psychological Corporation.

—— (1996) *Wechsler Objective Reading Dimensions.* Sidcup, Kent: Psychological Corporation.

Weinberg, W.A., Emslie, G.J. (1991) 'Attention deficit hyperactivity disorder: the differential diagnosis.' *Journal of Child Neurology*, **6** (Suppl.), S23–S36.

Whalen, C.K., Henker, B. (1991) 'Therapies for hyperactive children: comparisons, combinations and compromises.' *Journal of Consulting and Clinical Psychology*, **59**, 126–137.

Wolraich, M.L., Lindren, S., Stromquist, A., Milich, R., Davis, C., Watson, D. (1990) 'Stimulant medication use by primary care physicians in the treatment of attention deficit hyperactivity disorder.' *Pediatrics*, **86**, 95–101.

Woodward, L., Downey, L., Taylor, E. (1997) 'Child and family factors influencing the clinical referral of children with hyperactivity: a research note.' *Journal of Child Psychology and Psychiatry*, **38**, 479–485.

WHO (1988) *The ICD-10 Classification of Mental and Behavioural Disorders*. Geneva: World Health Organization.

Zagar, R., Bowers, N.D. (1983) 'The effect of time of day on problem-solving and classroom behavior.' *Psychology in Schools*, **20**, 337–345.

Zentall, S.S. (1986) 'Effects of color stimulation on performance and activity of hyperactive and nonhyperactive children.' *Journal of Educational Psychology*, **78**, 59–165.

APPENDIX 2.1
NEUROPSYCHOLOGICAL ASSESSMENTS OF ATTENTION/IMPULSIVITY

The continuous performance test (CPT), originally developed by Rosvold and colleagues (1956), is perhaps the most well-known measure of attention. There is no standard version of a CPT, but such tests generally are computerized and involve the repeated, rapid, visual or auditory presentation of stimuli (*e.g.* letters of the alphabet). The child is instructed to respond, usually by pressing a button, when a particular target stimulus (*e.g.* the letter 'X') or series of stimuli (*e.g.* the letter 'X' followed by the letter 'Y') appears. The task theoretically taps sustained attention, as vigilance over time is required for optimal performance. The actual length of the task can vary widely (*e.g.* 3–30 minutes).

Data provided by a CPT include number of targets missed (errors of omission) and time taken to respond to the targets (*i.e.* reaction time). Both of these measures are considered indicators of attentional processes. Responses to nontarget stimuli (errors of commission) can be construed as evidence of impulsivity. The CPT provides an opportunity to gather qualitative impressions on how a child responds to a boring, repetitive task that requires sustained attention and inhibition of inappropriate responses. Quantitative performance on a CPT should not be used to specifically diagnose children with attentional or hyperactivity problems (Matier-Sharma *et al.* 1995).

Paper and pencil cancellation tests provide an assessment of attention and are quite easy to administer. Again, there is no standard cancellation test, but the task generally involves presenting the child with a sheet of paper on which rows or arrays of letters or shapes are typed. The child is given a set amount of time to work and asked to read through the rows and tick off a predetermined target letter or shape each time they come across it. Data on number of target letters identified and missed, number of nontarget letters identified and total number processed in the allotted time are viewed as indicators of attention skills (Goodman and Stevenson 1989).

The Matching Familiar Figures Test (MFFT; Kagan 1966) is often used as a measure of impulsivity. Again, the primary use of the MFFT would be for developing a clinical picture of a child's cognitive tendencies, and not for diagnosing ADHD. The MFFT uses a matching-to-sample paradigm in which the child is shown a picture of a familiar object, then asked to scan six pictures and select the one that identically matches the sample. There are two versions of the MFFT, but the 20-item version is viewed as more reliable than the 12-item version (Cairns and Cammock 1978).

Pennington (1991) provides a review of the usefulness of other neuropsychological assessments in the evaluation of ADHD, including the Wisconsin Card Sorting Test, Tower of Hanoi, go–no-go tests, and the Rey Osterreith Complex Figure test.

3
AUTISM

Patricia Howlin

Background

Behavioural interventions for children with autism were first reported in the early 1960s (Hingtgen and Trost 1964, Wolf *et al.* 1964, Hewett 1965, Lovaas *et al.* 1966). The focus of these early studies was largely on the elimination of problem behaviours, such as self-injury or aggression, or on increasing particular areas of skill (such as rates of vocalization or the frequency of social responses). A combination of rewards (usually sweets and praise) and punishments (including the use of cattle prods and electric shocks) was used, but there was little attention to individual variables, or to environmental or other factors that might be responsible for causing or maintaining the child's behaviour. Intervention programmes were generally clinic-based, and the situations in which new behaviours were taught, or unwanted behaviours eliminated, frequently bore little or no relationship to the child's natural environment. In terms of language training, for example, it was recommended that: "To work most efficiently with a deviant child . . . the speech training should be carried out in a room containing as few distractions as possible" (Risley and Wolf 1967).

Typically, language programmes at that time concentrated on speech rather than wider aspects of communication. The child would work at a table on a one-to-one basis with the therapist, who, in order to increase vocalizations, would demonstrate a particular sound and then use physical prompts to ensure that the child formed the correct mouth and tongue movements. Praise and small items of food would be used to reward acceptable imitations. Once a single sound was established in this way, other sounds would be trained in a similar fashion. Sounds could then be paired together and used to identify items selected by the therapist. For example, if the child had learned to make the sounds 'K' and 'aah', s/he might then be prompted to combine these in an approximation to 'car'. Once an extensive naming vocabulary had been established, therapists would then often turn to published language 'packages' in order to enhance the level of grammatical structures used by the child.

These techniques were hailed as having a significant impact on language acquisition; some studies even claimed to have established 'near-normal speech' in less than a year (Marshall and Hegrenes 1970, Daley *et al.* 1972). As time went on, however, it became increasingly apparent that outcome was far from universally successful (for a review, see Howlin 1989). Lovaas (1977), for example, reported that over 90,000 trials were needed to teach one child just two simple word-approximations. Other, even less successful studies were presumably never reported in the literature at all.

Problems of maintenance and generalization also became increasingly apparent. The majority of these early intervention studies were conducted in specialist settings, with little or no parental involvement. Thus, even if improvements were reported, these often disappeared once the child was returned home (Lovaas *et al*. 1973). Subsequently, emphasis shifted to the use of school- and home-based programmes, with close liaison between parents and teachers becoming a central part of most successful interventions (Schopler and Reichler 1971, Hemsley *et al*. 1978, Short 1984, Howlin and Rutter 1987).

A more naturalistic approach to teaching and a focus on activities or materials that are of direct relevance to and of importance for the individual child are characteristic of recent programmes. By ensuring that the activities chosen are of interest to the child, and that the skills taught enhance immediate control over the environment, this in turn has led to a reduction in the need for 'artificial' rewards, such as sweets or food.

Factors underlying behaviour problems in autism

The range of behavioural difficulties associated with autism, and very many different ways of dealing with these, have been widely documented in both research and clinical literature. As with any other group of children, behaviours can be maintained or increased by the attention or reinforcement they elicit, and techniques such as time out, extinction or differential reinforcement can serve an important role in reducing unwanted behaviours, or establishing more desirable ones (see Emerson 1995). However, as is apparent from other chapters in this volume, they are by no means specific to the treatment of autism. The focus of this chapter, therefore, will be on understanding and dealing with the underlying causes of behavioural disturbances.

Although children with autism are frequently described as showing 'challenging behaviours', in fact, given the severity of their social and communication deficits and their need for ritual and routine, many could be considered to show far *fewer* challenges than might be expected. It is important to appreciate that, for much of their lives, they are expected to cope with a world in which they are able to understand almost nothing of what is happening around them; in which they are thrown daily into an ever-changing and unpredictable environment; where they lack even the rudimentary verbal skills necessary to make their needs known; and where they have no access to the internalized, imaginative facilities that are so crucial for dealing effectively with anxiety, uncertainty and distress. It is hardly surprising, therefore, that from time to time they resort to behaviours that can be difficult for other people to deal with. However, better understanding of the role that the fundamental social, communication and obsessional difficulties play in causing or maintaining problem behaviours can be of crucial importance in developing more effective strategies. Such understanding is also more likely to result in a focus on the need to improve functioning in these areas, rather than on the direct elimination of what may well be secondary problems. Table 3.1 indicates how the social and communication deficits found in autism, and the tendency towards ritualistic and stereotyped behaviours, can give rise to a range of different problems. Moreover, these problems are likely to vary according to the ability of any individual child.

Assessment for intervention

ENVIRONMENTAL AND PHYSICAL FACTORS

Before embarking on any treatment programme it is essential to carry out detailed assessments,

TABLE 3.1*
The principal diagnostic features of autism and their association with behaviour problems

Area of deficit	Associated problems	
	Less able children	More able children
Impairments in communication and understanding		
Inadequate language	Frustration, aggression; unacceptable attempts to control environment	Inappropriate use of speech (echolalia, verbal routines, obsessional questions, etc.)
Poor comprehension	Anxiety, distress and disruptive behaviours	Apparent lack of cooperation
Lack of internal language	No ability to play or occupy self	Poor imaginative skills; limited self-control
Impairments in social understanding		
Lack of social awareness	Withdrawal and isolation. Disturbed/disruptive and inappropriate behaviours in public	Attempts to socialize often inappropriate; may offend or antagonize others. Inability to 'read' others' feelings makes them appear insensitive, callous, even cruel
Obsessions and rituals		
Obsessional behaviour patterns	Can severely limit the acquisition of other more productive behaviours/skills	May involve other people in routines/rituals; can impose major limitations on other people's activities too
Disruption of routines	Can result in serious distress, disruption and aggression	
Dislike of change	Leads to very rigid and inflexible patterns of behaviour and great distress and anxiety if change is necessary	
Obsessional interests		May be pursued regardless of the consequences. Constant talk about these can antagonize others

*Reproduced by permission from Howlin (1998).

not only of the behaviours to be modified, but of the child as well. This is because apparently similar problems can have very different causes in different children, or within the same child at different times. For example, so-called 'aggressive' behaviours may result from a child's inability to communicate; because s/he lacks more effective strategies to control the environment; because of the attention such behaviours receive; because of frustration, distress or anxiety; or because of disruption to rituals and routines. Moreover, in many instances a combination of these variables may be operating. Pain or physical illness are other important factors to bear in mind, especially if there is a sudden upsurge in problems. For example, certain stereotyped and self-injurious behaviours have been found to follow minor illnesses including dermatitis and otitis media (Konstantareas and Homatidis 1987, Oliver 1995, Hall

1997). Gunsett *et al.* (1989) also stress the importance of carrying out medical screening before any psychological programmes are implemented, particularly in patients with no speech or with profound learning disabilities. They found that in a substantial number of such patients referred for self-injurious behaviours, there was some physical basis for the behaviour, including problems such as limb fractures, hernias, urinary tract infections, bowel problems, incorrect medication (especially anticonvulsants) and progressive brain deterioration.

COGNITIVE AND LINGUISTIC LEVELS

Assessments of children's cognitive and linguistic levels of functioning are also important, both for investigating the possible role that such difficulties may play in causing behaviour problems, and in devising appropriate intervention procedures. Dealing with the temper tantrums of a nonspeaking 4-year-old child with an IQ of 30, for example, will clearly require very different strategies to those that may be appropriate for a highly verbal 14-year-old with an 1Q of 130. Furthermore, informal observations, alone, can give quite misleading impressions of children's true intellectual ability. Children who appear alert and interested in their environment, or who have one or two isolated skills, may be mistakenly viewed as very intelligent. Those who are able to follow simple instructions (often only with accompanying gesture or other cues) may be described, quite erroneously, as "understanding every word you say", while children who have an extensive expressive vocabulary may actually have very limited comprehension skills. Conversely, some children whose speech is slow and halting, and who appear to show little interest in the activities around them, may be deemed as having severe learning difficulties when, in fact, many aspects of their cognitive development lie within the normal range.

Thus, standardized cognitive and linguistic assessments should be considered as a crucial prerequisite of any intervention programme. It is sometimes believed, because of the social and communication difficulties associated with autism, that traditional psychometric testing has little or no role to play in assessment. However, under the right conditions, and with appropriate materials, cognitive assessments of autistic children have been found to be just as valid and reliable as they are for other groups of children (Rutter 1985). A relatively brief formal assessment can reveal unsuspected areas of skill or deficit, which may be very relevant for intervention and which may not have been evident from unstructured observations alone. Information from standardized tests of language and cognition can also prove extremely useful in designing programmes to enhance particular areas of deficit (see Howlin 1998 for further details of appropriate assessments).

BEHAVIOURAL VARIABLES

Traditional behavioural therapy tended to take a somewhat simplistic 'ABC' approach to the analysis of behavioural problems. Following precise delineation of the *B*ehaviour to be modified, attempts would be made to identify, and subsequently to alter the *A*ntecedents and the *C*onsequences of that behaviour. However, in the case of many children with autism, it can be extremely difficult to establish, with any degree of certainty, what the antecedents or the consequences of the behaviour may be. Moreover, a focus on the observed behaviour does not necessarily lead to the most appropriate form of treatment (Emerson and Bromley

1995). For example, a child might begin to self-injure in a particular setting because s/he has been reminded of an earlier (but no longer existing) distressing occurrence, that had previously ceased when self-injury commenced. In such a case, direct observations will be of little use in identifying the relevant variables.

Because the observed *form* of a challenging behaviour may give few clues as to its real role, recent intervention studies have focused instead on the *function* or 'message' of that behaviour. The aim is to establish what it achieves for all the individuals concerned (carers as well as children) and to explore the alternative behaviours that might be encouraged to replace it (Sturmey 1996).

THE FUNCTIONAL ANALYSIS OF BEHAVIOUR

Recent experimental studies of the 'challenging' behaviours shown by children with autism have consistently demonstrated that many such behaviours serve an important communicative function (Durand 1990). Indeed, analyses of these behaviours suggest that they may sometimes be the only way in which a child with limited linguistic abilities can rapidly, effectively and predictably control her/his environment.

Five main functions of aggressive, self-injurious, stereotyped or other disruptive behaviours have been identified (Durand and Crimmins 1988, Durand and Carr 1991). These are: (1) to indicate the need for help or attention; (2) to escape from stressful situations or activities; (3) to obtain desired objects; (4) to protest against unwanted events/activities; (5) to obtain stimulation.

If the primary function of a behaviour can be identified it is then possible to provide the child with alternative means to obtain the same ends. The choice of strategy taught will depend on the child's cognitive and linguistic ability, but might range from teaching her/him to push a button, lever or switch, or to use signs, symbols, pictures, words or even simple phrases (such as "Help me"). As long as the newly acquired behaviour has a rapid and predictable impact on the child's environment this can result in significant reductions in undesirable behaviours (Durand and Carr 1991).

Despite the potential practical significance of this approach to intervention, it is important to be aware that the majority of studies have been conducted in highly staffed experimental settings. Detailed analyses of the possible functions of undesirable behaviours may require considerable time, expertise and technology and are often impracticable within school- or home-based settings. Functional analysis certainly is not as easy as ABC (Owens and MacKinnon 1993). Moreover, it may be much more difficult to identify the factors maintaining a particular behaviour than some of the earlier literature would seem to indicate. Emerson and Bromley (1995) failed to identify any specific function for challenging behaviours in around 25 per cent of cases, and a third of behaviours appeared to be influenced by multiple factors. Hall (1997), in a very sophisticated assessment of self-injurious and stereotyped behaviours in 16 children with severe to profound learning disabilities, was able to identify a consistent underlying function for self-injury in only four cases and for stereotyped behaviours in only six cases. Moreover, knowledge about the variables maintaining one class of behaviours may not necessarily be of any value in predicting the behavioural function underlying other forms of challenging behaviour shown by the same individual.

It is also necessary to bear in mind that, despite the evident success of this approach in many cases, there have been few if any randomized control studies. Most have been multiple baseline, single case or small group reports, and although those that have been published are certainly encouraging, there is no way of ascertaining how many unsuccessful studies may also have been conducted.

Nevertheless, it seems that this approach to assessment and treatment can play a major role in reducing problem behaviours. Interest in these methods has also led to the development of a number of rating scales or questionnaires that can be used, within the home or school, to help identify the possible functions of disruptive behaviours (see Sturmey 1996). Probably the most widely used of these is the Motivation Assessment Scale designed by Durand and Crimmins (1988). This attempts to classify behaviour into four main categories: attention seeking; self-stimulatory; escape or avoidance; or as indicating the need for help or assistance. However, there are concerns about the reliability and validity of this scale when used in naturalistic settings, and, more importantly, the four summary categories cannot encompass all the possible reasons for disruptive behaviours. In particular, they cannot identify idiosyncratic or multifunctional causes (Sturmey 1995).

Increasing communicative skills

Although there are certainly major problems in identifying all the possible causes of 'challenging' behaviours, it has become increasingly clear over recent years that impairments in communication and understanding frequently play a significant role. Schuler *et al.* (1989) have developed a relatively simple questionnaire that can be used by parents or teachers systematically to explore how the child expresses her/his need to do something (sit by someone, get attention, obtain food or other object, protest if something is taken away, etc.). This process can again help to indicate how behaviours that are often viewed as 'inappropriate' (screaming, self-injury, tantrums, aggression, etc.) can have important communicative functions. Such information can then be used to plan ways in which alternative and more acceptable responses might be established. Moreover, by helping carers to appreciate that such behaviours may be a function of poor *communication* skills, rather than being 'deliberate' acts of aggression or provocation, this approach can also have a very positive effect on other people's attitudes and responses towards the child.

In a slightly different format is the interview protocol devised by Finnerty and Quill (1991). This uses many of the items in the Schuler schedule, but questions are grouped into 26 communicative functions, with sample scenarios provided to guide the interview. The interview describes a situation that is likely to encourage some form of communication. For example, to assess how the child obtains attention, the interviewee is asked "You are giving your attention to another child: what does X do [or say, in the case of a verbal child]?". Descriptions of the child's verbal or nonverbal responses can then be collated, and this approach can be used to summarize the child's communicative skills in several different areas (Quill 1995).

Follow-up studies indicate that most children with autism who have not developed useful speech by the age of 6 or 7 years remain very impaired in their ability to communicate verbally. For them, some form of alternative communication system will be required, and the appropriate choice of system will depend on the child's particular pattern of skills and disabilities. Layton and Watson (1995), for example, provide a useful breakdown of the different skills required for using signs, pictures or written words.

Sign systems, especially those developed for use with children with learning disabilities, have been widely used to augment communication skills. The Makaton system (Walker 1980), is extensively used in schools in the UK. This has several different levels of complexity, and now incorporates symbols as well as signs, but in the early stages the 'vocabulary' is characterized by signs that are very simple, concrete, and require the use of only one hand.

The main advantage of signs is that they can be more easily shaped and prompted than speech, and there is little doubt that the use of signs has enabled large numbers of children who were previously without language to communicate somewhat more effectively. However, in the case of children with autism, the evidence to show that communication can be significantly enhanced in this way is limited. Kiernan (1983), reviewing the outcome of signing programmes found that these were very variable. After two to three years, some children had acquired an extensive signing vocabulary (400 sign combinations) or had begun to use speech, whereas others had managed to learn only one or two signs. Other studies indicate that problems of generalization and maintenance are similar to those experienced in verbal training programmes. The communicative use of signs may also remain very limited. Thus, Attwood *et al.* (1988) found that the signing of children with autism was very similar to their use of spoken language—*i.e.* it was stereotyped, repetitive, and used mainly to achieve the child's immediate goals. Signing was rarely used to share experiences, to express feelings or emotions, or to communicate in a reciprocal and spontaneous fashion.

Clinical experience also suggests that many children prefer to use the most 'telegraphic' style of signing that they can get away with, and although this may be understood by familiar adults, it is hardly likely to enhance general communication. Multipurpose signs such as 'Please' are probably best avoided, since children rapidly learn that only the one gesture is needed to obtain anything from toys, food or cuddles to a visit to the lavatory.

A further problem related to signing is the fact that the majority of people in the child's environment will not know how to sign, and will therefore be unable to respond to her/his attempts to communicate. Although exposure to signing is highly related to outcome, often the only people who can sign with or to the child are parents or teachers. Konstantareas (1987) found that the amount of adult involvement was significantly related to the level of signing acquired by the child, but of course most parents and teachers tend to use signs far less frequently than they do speech.

On the whole, a pictorially based system makes least demand on cognitive, linguistic or memory skills, although, again, it is essential that the pictures or photographs used reflect the individual's particular interests or needs. It also seems to be important for the child to take an *active role* in using and handling such materials (*e.g.* using Velcro or stickers to indicate the activities completed, or to be done, rather than looking passively at charts constructed by others). The Picture Exchange Communication System (PECS) of Bondy and Frost (1996), which involves the child presenting picture cards which are then exchanged for the desired object or activity, is an example of this type of system.

If the child has learned to use or respond to pictures without difficulty, it may then be possible to progress to symbol systems, which are more flexible and also allow the construction of simple phrases. Recent developments in computer software (*e.g.* Boardmaker or Picture Communication Systems*) mean that it is now possible to create large numbers of different symbols quickly and early. These can be automatically scaled to the right size to use in books or wall charts, or as overlays for computer keyboards. Like pictures, symbols require only minimal motor skill on the part of the user and are easily understood by untrained observers.

Once the association between the activity/object and picture/symbol/chart is established, individualized sets of photographs, pictures or symbols can be used to increase both communication and understanding (Quill 1995). Whatever system is chosen, this must be readily available to the child and her/his carers at all times. Possible ways of ensuring easy access are to have the picture/symbol/word sets on cards in a simple 'Filofax'-type system, attached to the child's belt, in a hip bag, or worn, like an identity badge, on a chain. Materials also need to be strongly bound and quickly replaceable. Equipment that is forever getting lost or torn is of little use to anyone.

Computerized communicative devices have become steadily more sophisticated in recent years. Some are now specially designed for children with autism, in that they have a specific focus on turn-taking and reciprocal interaction. Interchangeable keyboards of increasing complexity make it possible for children to progress gradually from single symbol boards (*e.g.* with a large red square or circle that will emit a sound to attract attention) to, eventually, the independent use of multisymbol displays that are personally tailored to the individual's own environment, needs or interests. Computers can also of course be very valuable general teaching aids for more able children who may respond better to visually than to verbally presented material. However, when using computers with this group, care needs to be taken to ensure that some social interaction is also required, otherwise an obsession with the technology may take over.

Some parents understandably express concerns that, by focusing on alternative forms of communication, this will minimize the chances of their child ever learning to speak. However, developing competence in the use of signs or symbols may actually encourage some previously nonverbal children to use speech (Kiernan 1983, Yoder and Layton 1988, Howlin 1989), while for those who do not, it is crucial to establish an effective and socially acceptable form of communication as early as possible. (For further discussion of ways to enhance communicative functioning in nonverbal children, see Schuler *et al.* 1997, Wetherby *et al.* 1997.)

IMPROVING COMMUNICATION IN CHILDREN WHO CAN TALK
Although around half of all children with autism develop some functional use of speech (Lord and Rutter 1994), even amongst those with a good expressive vocabulary there are often persisting and pervasive impairments in spoken language, and in understanding complex or abstract concepts.

For younger children, who are able to use some words or sounds spontaneously,

*Mayer-Johnson Co., Solana Beach, CA, USA.

individualized language programmes are important for improving comprehension, increasing the complexity of speech, or correcting problems of intonation or articulation. However, it is essential that such programmes are aimed at a level that is appropriate to the child's cognitive and linguistic development and that the structures or concepts involved are ones that are of direct relevance to the child (see Prizant *et al.* 1997). Language cannot be taught in brief, one hour speech therapy sessions, but language therapists can play a crucial role in ensuring that all those living and working with the child use effective and consistent strategies to encourage speech, develop imaginative skills and improve understanding. Descriptive assessments of the way in which children use and understand language, such as the Pragmatics Profile of Early Communication Skills (which is based on a structured parental interview—Dewart and Summers 1988) or the Social Use of Language Programme (Rinaldi 1992) can also be used to provide guidelines for improving receptive and conversational skills. As long as the words taught are of practical value to the child, in that they allow her/him immediate access to desired objects or activities, then artificial rewards should not be needed. Indeed there is evidence that the unnecessary introduction of extrinsic reinforcers may actually interfere with learning (Howlin and Rutter 1987).

It is also important to be aware that children with no *apparent* language difficulties may require some augmentative communication systems from time to time. Almost all children with autism, no matter how able, have difficulties with abstract language or in dealing with complex sequences of instructions. Thus, although they may understand the *individual words* spoken, they may well misinterpret or fail to understand the underlying meaning of what is said. If told, in an art class, to "Paint the child sitting next to you" they may well do exactly that, and then have no idea why they have got into trouble. In such circumstances it is essential that the speaker makes sure that the words used really do convey what is meant— *i.e.* "Paint a *picture* of the child sitting next to you."

When the task requirements are more complex (such as having to complete activities in a set order, as in following a recipe), checklists of simple instructions, picture or cartoon sequences of the activities to be completed, or symbols designating the tasks to be done can all help greatly to improve cooperation. Again, the reward should lie in the successful completion of the task, not in unrelated activities.

Perhaps the best known example of a very successful, visually based instructional system is the TEACCH educational programme, initially developed in North Carolina (Schopler *et al.* 1995). This relies heavily on visual cues or 'jigs', so that, throughout the child's school day, different coloured work areas or different coloured containers are used to indicate where the child should be, what s/he should be doing, where work should begin or be placed when finished, and even where to play. However, as with any treatment package, it is important that the basic components are adapted to suit the needs of the individual and her/his environment. It is also important to plan for the gradual reduction of such cues if the child is eventually to be able to function in less structured surroundings (Jordan and Powell 1995).

REPETITIVE AND STEREOTYPED SPEECH
Although echolalia is often considered as inappropriate and noncommunicative, as well as

sometimes being extremely irritating, careful analysis indicates that it frequently serves an important communicative function (Prizant and Schuler 1987, Rydell and Prizant 1995). As with any other 'autistic' behaviour, it is crucial to assess the role that the echolalia serves before attempts are made to modify this.

Echoing may be an indication of children's lack of understanding; it may be important in helping them to consolidate what others say, as well as providing them with the opportunity to practise new words or expressions. Moreover, in that echolalia is likely to increase when children are distressed or anxious, it may signify that they are experiencing undue pressure (Rydell and Mirenda 1994). Repetition can also play a role in rehearsing potentially worrying situations, in dealing with feelings of anger, or in helping to allay anxiety. Greater understanding of why such behaviours may occur, and recognition of the potential importance of these, should lead to more appropriate intervention strategies, with a focus on altering the factors causing the echolalia, rather than on the symptom itself.

Taking appropriate steps to ensure that instructions or questions are fully understood (by simplifying the language used, or supplementing this with pictures, written instructions or other cues), can significantly reduce stereotyped and echolalic speech (Rydell and Prizant 1995). Repetitive questioning (which often tends to escalate the more adults respond to it), may also be reduced by directing the child to charts, pictures, calendars or lists, which provide her/him with the required information in a more permanent form. Sonia, for example, was a 13-year-old girl with an obsession with petrol stations. She was allowed to go with the school bus every Friday to have it filled with diesel, but every day, particularly as the week progressed, she would anxiously interrogate staff about what day it was, and when she would be allowed to go to the petrol station. A weekly chart, illustrating clearly the activities for each day and culminating with a photo of the bus and petrol pumps, was drawn up and whenever the obsessional questioning began Sonia was sent off to look at her chart. Fascination with the photograph of the petrol station, as well as the clear visual information that the chart displayed, helped greatly to diminish both her anxiety and her repetitive and intrusive questioning.

Dealing with unnecessary stress, by supplying the child with adequate help in cognitively or socially demanding situations, may also have a considerable impact. Minimizing disruption to daily routine, and ensuring that daily life is as predictable and as consistent as possible, and that necessary changes are predicted well in advance can all help to decrease the frequency of repetitive speech.

Stereotyped speech (*e.g.* bombarding visitors with questions about the make of their car, or lengthy monologues about the lighting systems on particular railway networks) may be an indication that, although the child wishes to make social contact, s/he lacks the necessary conversational skills. Again, help to initiate and cope with basic conversational exchanges—perhaps by utilizing role-play or drama techniques—is often the most effective way of addressing problems of this kind.

Of course, sometimes, stereotyped speech may be used deliberately because of the attention it generates. Repetitive phrases, swearing or other provocative utterances often provoke a rapid response from adults and other children and are all too easily reinforced. In such cases, as well as increasing the child's repertoire of appropriate speech, strategies involving extinction (ignoring) or 'time out' (removal of ongoing rewards) may be necessary. Howlin and Rutter (1987), for example, describe the strategies used to reduce deliberately provocative remarks by a 7-year-old boy. Living in very cramped, inadequate conditions his mother struggled against the odds to keep the house and children as clean and orderly as possible. His most effective way of getting her attention was to describe every thing as 'dirty'. Physical punishment had no effect, and recognizing this, his mother eventually learned to ignore these remarks. From time to time he would try out new and equally annoying phrases, but after an initial reaction his mother managed to ignore these too. The frequency of such remarks declined rapidly and they were eventually overcome entirely when his mother encouraged him to *write them* rather than say them.

Such techniques, if used *consistently*, can have a rapid and positive effect on behaviour— the problem lies in being consistent. Thus, swearing or other abusive language may be relatively easy to ignore by parents who are relaxed and in control. After a sleepless night, when under stress, or in conditions where they have little control (*e.g.* in church, on the top of a bus, or in a supermarket queue) it can be almost impossible not to respond. Intermittent reinforcement of this kind can actually result in an increase in unwanted behaviour, and hence extinction programmes, although highly effective *in principle*, can prove much more difficult to implement in practice. Parents also need to be given support during the early stages of such programmes when the 'extinction burst' (an initial increase in the behaviour when reinforcement is first withdrawn) is likely to occur.

IMPROVING OTHERS' COMMUNICATION SKILLS
Although, with appropriate help and encouragement, children with autism may show improvements in both their use and understanding of language, the communication deficit is central to the disorder and no amount of therapy will overcome this entirely. Much can be achieved, however, by making the adults in the child's environment more attentive to the language that they themselves use. Instructions should be simple and concise, and every attempt made to ensure that the words used actually mean what they say. Metaphor, slang, irony or colloquialisms are all best avoided: one young girl refused ever to enter a swimming pool again having been told by her teacher, "Make sure you dry yourself properly, or your clothes will stick to you." Even vague concepts such as "Perhaps", I'll think about it", or "We'll see" are liable to produce confusion and anxiety. If the child is required to do some-thing, an unambiguous request such as "Go and get your coat" will be more productive than a phrase such as "Can you get your coat?" (which might well be answered in the affirmative but without resulting in any action). Questions also need to be carefully worded. One little boy, whose visit to the lavatory seemed rather prolonged, was asked by his concerned teacher, "Do you need a hand?". "No thankyou," came the polite reply from behind the door, "there's plenty of paper in here." Other apparently minor changes in wording can have surprising effects. One girl's severe distress at being told, before a trip to France, that she would be "going to sleep on the train" changed to pleasure and relief when this was altered to "going to bed in the train".

Unfortunately, predicting in advance what particular turn of phrase is likely to give rise to problems is very much a matter of trial and error. However, whenever a request is not complied with, or if a statement meets with an upsurge in echolalia, irritation or anxiety, the speaker should first assume that what s/he has said has been misunderstood or misinterpreted. Simplifying or changing the words that are used may have a much greater impact than attempts to modify the child's response. Once again, the value of written or pictorial cues to augment the words used cannot be over-emphasized.

Ameliorating social difficulties

The social impairment in autism affects almost every aspect of the child's functioning, whatever her/his intellectual ability. In children who are more severely disabled, highly inappropriate behaviours, such as screaming, undressing or masturbating in public may be a major cause of disturbance. In the case of those who are more able, the problems tend to be much more subtle and include impairments in empathy, social understanding, or reciprocity and synchronization (*i.e.* saying or doing things that in themselves are not unacceptable, but at the wrong time, in the wrong place or with the wrong person).

Parents of older children with autism also tend to become more concerned, not by their social *isolation* but rather their lack of social inhibition. A number of examples, taken from clinical practice, illustrate the potential dangers of this:

- Sally, a 14-year-old, would strip off her clothing any time she met anyone new, in order to show them her appendix scar.

- Daniel, an 8-year-old with an obsession for excavating machines, would spend all his free time on building sites and took any opportunity to gain access to the cab of 'diggers'.

- William, a 13-year-old with a fascination for rugby, would wander in and out of players' changing rooms, chatting to them as if he had known them all his life.

- Gillian, a 15-year-old with an obsession for certain makes of wrist watch, would approach strangers, roll up their sleeves and then follow them if they were wearing her favourite make.

- Suzie, a pubescent 12-year-old, still insists on wearing very childish clothes (ankle socks and very short dresses). She has a tendency to develop intense 'crushes' on male neighbours or school teachers, insisting on cuddling them and sitting on their lap.

In such cases, it is clearly the need to discourage rather than encourage social initiations that presents problems.

In many ways, the more obvious social problems of children with severe cognitive impairments are often easier to deal with. Firm and consistent guidance is needed, from the outset, about what behaviours are or are not acceptable. If, as a small child, there are clear and invariable rules—such as never undressing or masturbating in public, and not touching strangers or their belongings—and if the child also learns that disruptive behaviour in response to such prohibitions results in the cessation of more pleasurable activities, then these behaviours are much less likely to give rise to problems in later childhood. Children with autism are, by definition, somewhat rigid in their behaviour patterns, and if acceptable behaviours are established when they are very young these are likely to be maintained. The converse, of course, is also true, so that once unacceptable behaviours take hold, they will be very difficult to shift in later years, especially as the child grows bigger. Parents, however, may need a great deal of help and support during these early years if they are to develop effective management strategies. Young children with autism are clearly often deeply disturbed and confused, and most parents, unwilling to increase their distress, will tend to give in to many of their demands. Helping parents to understand when it is acceptable or necessary to say "No" and to recognize when consistency is crucial can help to avoid future problems. Removing a screaming 3-year-old from a shop, because he insists on stripping off all his clothes is embarrassing enough; attempts to remove a 13-year-old in the same circumstances will prove far more difficult.

It is also important that parents are aware of behaviours which, although not necessarily inappropriate in a young child, may become progressively more unacceptable as s/he grows older. A young girl who warmly hugs and kisses everyone she meets, or a little boy who loves the feel of women's tights may be treated with fond indulgence; the same behaviours in older teenagers or adults will provoke a very different response. Difficulties in social understanding and awareness mean that the child with autism will either be impervious to other peoples' changed reactions or be totally confused by the fact that behaviours that were once tolerated, even encouraged, are suddenly deemed to be 'wrong'. On the whole, it is far preferable to introduce simple and invariable rules (you only kiss people in the family; you can only touch mummy's tights) that may be relaxed in later years if necessary, than to have initially very loose guidelines, which suddenly have to be made more restrictive. A toddler who has been allowed to take off all his clothes whenever he wanted, will find it very difficult to change this behaviour when he begins attending school. On the other hand, a child who has only ever been allowed to take her clothes off in the home can be taught, as she grows older, that it may be acceptable to remove her clothes in other *specified* situations, such as the family doctor's surgery.

The major problem, here, is that social behaviour is not governed by simple rules; if such rules do exist they are highly complex and constantly changing according to the social context. Nevertheless, as far as the child with autism is concerned it is preferable to have consistent (if sometimes inadequate) rules, than no rules at all.

It is dealing with more complex and subtle social deficits that presents much more of a challenge. Knowing how to make friends, recognizing what other people are feeling or thinking, and reacting appropriately, are fundamental human aptitudes; they are not rule-based skills that are acquired through teaching. Thus, interventions designed to overcome such basic deficits are almost certain to be limited in their effectiveness. There is some evidence that social skills groups specifically designed for children or adolescents with autism can improve certain aspects of social functioning (Mesibov 1984, Williams 1989), but on the whole generalization to untrained settings tends to be limited. Social skills training is best conducted in each and every situation to which the child is exposed, so that s/he learns how to respond appropriately at home, with relatives, in shops, at school, or with the peer group. Each of these situations will require different social strategies, and teaching *in situ* is far more likely to be effective than teaching in the relative isolation of a social skills group.

Learning how to interact appropriately with children of their own age is often one of the most difficult and demanding tasks for a child with autism. The 'rules' of engagement—

of knowing how to enter a group of children, how to join in with their activities, how to talk to them—are all highly complex, unwritten, and generally poorly understood (Dodge *et al.* 1983), and hence almost impossible to teach. Because of this, some researchers have shifted the focus of attention onto nonautistic peers, systematically teaching them to play and interact more effectively with the child with autism (Wolfberg and Schuler 1993, Lord 1995). Roeyers (1996) has also shown that simply providing non-disabled peers with information about children with autism and general instructions about ways to encourage them to play, can improve the frequency and style of joint interactions. Programmes of this kind can result in important short-term gains and are clearly important for improving opportunities for integration. Nevertheless, they do require skilled input from teachers if the interactions are to be effective, and it can prove difficult, even if very generous reinforcement programmes are used, to maintain peers' cooperation over the longer term (Lord 1984).

Other recent approaches to the treatment of social problems have focused on more fundamental deficits in 'theory of mind'. The inability of children with autism to 'mind-read', *i.e.* to understand other people's beliefs, ideas, thoughts or feelings, has received much attention over recent years (see Baron Cohen 1995). A number of studies have found that even after relatively brief training programmes involving computers, pictures, photographs, toys or actors, children with autism do show improvements in their ability to understand beliefs and emotions (Ozonoff and Miller 1995, Hadwin *et al.* 1996, Swettenham 1996). Not unexpectedly, given the brevity and circumscribed nature of such programmes, generalization to other, untrained aspects of 'theory of mind' is poor. Nevertheless, even this limited success suggests that teaching packages specifically designed to increase the ability to 'mind-read' could be an important and valuable addition to the educational curriculum for many children with autism (Howlin *et al.* 1998). [For a more detailed discussion of approaches to dealing with social difficulties, see Quill (1995) and Howlin (1998).]

Coping with stereotyped and ritualistic behaviours
Ritualistic and stereotyped behaviours are a further major cause of problems in autism. Many different ways of dealing with these problems have been reported in the literature, but generally it seems that a 'graded change' approach to intervention is the most effective. For a child with autism, repetitive, ritualistic activities often play a crucial role in reducing anxiety or in providing them with some control over what is otherwise a very confusing and unpredictable world (see Jolliffe *et al.* 1992). If an attempt is made suddenly to restrict or prohibit such behaviours, this can lead to unacceptably high levels of anxiety and distress, and because of the resulting disturbance most parents quickly give in. Moreover, without careful planning, children may well develop replacement rituals or routines that prove even more disruptive.

In order to maintain parental cooperation and consistency, it is generally more effective to modify the behaviour *gradually* until it no longer interferes with the child's or the family's other activities. Howlin and Rutter (1987) describe a variety of strategies that can be used to reduce stereotyped and ritualistic behaviours. However, the crucial goals are to minimize anxiety and distress (for both parents and child); to aim for gradual but achievable behavioural

TABLE 3.2
Stages in setting limits on a 3-year-old boy's obsession with Thomas The Tank Engine trains

1. Picture calendar, indicating when access to 'Thomas' videos and train sets is allowed, produced by parents
2. Videos made unavailable before school; 'Thomas' book read over breakfast instead
3. Videos restricted to one per evening after school; weekend access unrestricted; unlimited access to train sets
4. Limits on 'Thomas' clothing imposed; school agree that no 'Thomas' clothes can be worn there. No restrictions at home
5. Access to 'Thomas' train sets gradually restricted by increasing alternative activities (including 'Thomas' books, board games, etc.)
6. New electric train set provided at home; allowed in conjunction with some 'Thomas' toys; but not train sets
7. 'Thomas' trains moved to grandmother's house; access only available at weekends. Interests in trains, generally, encouraged

change, rather than dramatic improvements; to weigh up the potential advantages, as well as obvious disadvantages, of the obsession, and wherever possible to capitalize on these.

The following guidelines seem to be particularly helpful.

(1) *Intervene early:* rituals, routines or preoccupations that appear quite harmless when the child is small can easily become far less acceptable as individuals become larger and more determined to carry them out.

For example, one young child had a relatively innocuous fascination with watching people's washing machines. Family, friends and neighbours were happy to encourage this, but by the time he was 17 he was in constant trouble with the police for breaking into property in order to indulge his obsession.

The intensity of such behaviours can also increase to unacceptable levels over time. Understandably, the bewildered parents of a young infant tend to give in to the screams or tantrums that can occur because they have taken the 'wrong' route, or have tried to change the way in which a task is completed. Over the years, however, the child's demands may become increasingly draconian, until parents find themselves trapped in a web of complex and elaborate routines.

(2) *Establish clear and consistent rules* for: *Where and When* the activity is permitted; *Who* it can be carried out with; and *How long* it can go on for.

This ensures that the child knows not only when the behaviour is not permitted but also when it is allowed.

Table 3.2 presents an example of how one child's overwhelming preoccupation with Thomas the Tank Engine trains was gradually overcome. By the time he was barely 3 years old, his parents realized that the obsession was becoming so pervasive that they had to intervene in some way. At that age their son would wear only Thomas the Tank Engine clothes, spent all his time watching or reenacting Thomas videos, and talked of almost nothing else.

(3) *Ensure that change is introduced one step at a time*, so that any distress to the child is kept to a minimum. Setting very small goals also optimizes the chance of long-term success.

Amanda, for example, ate an extremely limited range of foods and also insisted that these were of a particular brand. She would eat only at a certain time, sit only in one place at the table, accepted only specific items of china and cutlery, and insisted that each item of food be in a particular position on the plate. To complicate the situation still further, she demanded that her father sat throughout the meal with his feet crossed in a certain way. Her parents began by slightly altering the time of meals. She was told the meal would be on the table between 11.50 and 12.10, but that it would not be exactly at 12.00, as she had previously insisted. Gradually, the variety of plates from which she would eat was increased and her place moved slightly at the table. Finally, if she did not stare at her father's feet throughout the meal, she was rewarded with a favourite video. Mealtimes remain somewhat rigid affairs, but at least they are less fraught and other members of the family are no longer involved in her routines.

(4) *Explore possible underlying factors.* High levels of stereotyped or repetitive behaviour are often an indication of uncertainty, anxiety or distress.

Such problems can be significantly reduced by ensuring that the child's daily programme is predictable, and appropriately stimulating and structured.

(5) *Consider possible environmental modifications*, and, if necessary, reduce unnecessary demands on the child, encourage more flexible attitudes in adults, or make relatively simple modifications to the daily routine or environment.

In mainstream schools, for example, many children with autism become very distressed (and hence more ritualistic) if they are forced to take part in group games or 'join in' at play times, or when they have to scramble to find somewhere to sit at the start of each lesson. Allowing children to avoid such socially demanding situations, letting them spend play/game times in the library or carrying out other tasks, or providing them with a set place in which to sit, may, again, have much greater impact than a complex behavioural programme.

(6) *Help children to cope with change.* Although a structured and settled daily programme is essential for progress, it is neither possible nor productive to avoid change completely. Fortunately, in many cases it is *unpredictable* change that causes most difficulties.

Thus, the solution is to ensure that the child is fully aware of what is going to happen at any time. Since verbal explanations are rarely adequate, visual representations (in the form of picture calendars, symbols or written lists) of forthcoming activities, or of alterations to the regular routine, are most likely to be effective. In Samantha's case, for example, any unpredictable alterations could give rise to major disturbance. If a teacher's car was not in the parking area when she arrived at school, or if the person supervising the school crossing had changed, the remainder of the day's activities would be totally disrupted. Increasing her awareness, in advance, of possible changes helped to reduce these problems. Picture calendars were used to illustrate the next days' activities, and photographs of staff members were used to indicate who would be at school and who would be away. If, as often happened, a teacher was away without prior warning, staff would focus on helping Samantha to find the appropriate photo and place it in the 'Away Today' column.

(7) *Make use of obsessions.* Although it may sometimes be necessary to eliminate certain ritualistic activities entirely, on the whole, once an acceptable level of control is reached, stereotyped behaviours and interests can have many positive features.

They may serve as extremely powerful reinforcers for developing more productive activities and may well minimize the need for other forms of reinforcement (Howlin and Rutter 1987, Koegel and Koegel 1995). Problems of satiation are far less likely to occur. They may also be an essential source of comfort or self-occupation for a child with few other interests or abilities. Follow-up studies suggest, too, that if obsessional skills and interests are appropriately encouraged and developed they can play a crucial role in later social and educational integration (Kanner 1973).

Early, intensive behavioural programmes

There is little doubt that the use of behaviourally based interventions has had a major impact on the lives of very many children with autism and their families. It is also clear from research into early therapeutic and educational programmes that progress tends to be greater if children are involved from as young an age as possible (preferably before 4 years of age— Rogers 1996). On the whole, however, behavioural programmes have been viewed as a means of ameliorating the problems associated with autism, rather than as a potential 'cure'. Nevertheless, over recent years, the intensive early intervention programme of Lovaas and his colleagues (Lovaas 1993, 1996; McEachin et al. 1993; Perry et al. 1995) is said to have resulted in 42 per cent of children with autism maintaining "normal functioning at follow-up" (average age of 11.5 years). Intervention, which is home-based, takes place for 40 hours per week and lasts from around the age of 2 to 4 years (Lovaas 1996). These claims have aroused criticism because of possible biases in subject selection, problems of research design and, most importantly, in the definitions of 'normality' used (Schopler et al. 1989, Rutter 1996). Thus, children are claimed to have 'recovered' if they are of normal IQ and can be assimilated into mainstream education. Since around 20 per cent of all autistic children are of normal intellectual ability, and many attend mainstream schools despite showing the characteristic triad of impairments, such criteria cannot be used as evidence of normal or even near-normal functioning (Mesibov 1993).

From a practical point of view, too, this approach poses many problems. The cost in emotional, financial or practical terms is clearly very high and may well prove too much for many parents. Moreover, although programmes of this kind may enhance short-term progress there is little to show that the benefits last beyond childhood, or that they extend to the family as a whole. Satisfactory, independent evaluations are still required (Rutter 1996), but were the claims to be substantiated this could lead to major changes in the ways in which treatment is currently provided and funded.

Other approaches to intervention

There are of course many other approaches to the treatment of autism, and the fact that some children do show substantial improvements as they grow older has led to claims that particular treatments can significantly affect outcome, or even bring about a 'cure'. Among such interventions are 'holding' therapy (Welch 1988, Richer and Zappella 1989); 'facilitated communication' (Biklen 1993); music therapy (Trevarthen et al. 1996); scotopic sensitivity training, which involves the wearing of specialist spectacles (Irlen 1995); auditory integration, which focuses on desensitization to sounds of particular frequencies (Stehli 1992; Rimland

and Edelson 1994, 1995). Various vitamin and drug treatments have also been claimed to improve many of the basic deficits associated with autism. In particular, fenfluramine and more recently certain selective serotonin uptake inhibitors (fluoxetine and fluvoxamine— Lewis 1996, McDougle *et al.* 1996) have been recommended as a means of reducing autistic symptomatology more generally.

A variety of teaching approaches have also been promoted as having a significant impact on outcome. These include the Japanese-originated 'Daily Life Therapy', with its focus on highly structured, physically oriented programmes, practised in the Higashi schools (see Gould *et al.* 1991 for details). The 'Options' method of Kaufman (1981), which relies on therapists participating in the child's ritualistic and obsessional behaviours in order to foster social contacts, also claims dramatic results (for a detailed review of different therapies, see Howlin 1998).

Unfortunately, few if any of these claims are supported by adequate experimental data and, to date, there is no good evidence that any cures for autism exist. Many able children do well despite totally inadequate provision, and to a great extent eventual outcome is dependent on innate cognitive, linguistic and social abilities. Before parents succumb to the temptation of parting from large amounts of money, or in some cases (as in specialist boarding school provision) from their own child, they should try to obtain as much information as possible, not only about the children for whom the treatment has worked but also about the characteristics of those for whom it has been less successful. Claims that the treatment works equally well for all need to be treated with particular caution. Parents need to enquire whether treatment seems to work better with older or younger children; for those with or without language; or for those who are more, or less, cognitively able. They should be encouraged to find out what sort of assessments are carried out prior to treatment and what methods (other than selective anecdotal reports) have been used to assess outcome. They also need accurate information about what happens to other children with autism as they grow older, so that reported outcomes following treatment can be judged in the light of what might be expected in the absence of any special treatments. Before jumping headlong into therapy, families should be helped, too, to weigh up the overall cost of treatment; the amount of time that will be involved; any foreseeable pressures or restrictions on other aspects of family life; and the possible impact on the child of having to cope with major change, or even separation from the family. Finally, they should also be offered detailed information on local facilities, support groups, educational provision and so forth. These are unlikely to have been widely advertized or to have featured in the national press, but may well be able to provide families and children with much needed and sometimes highly effective help. If parents are better informed of what is available within their own area, they may find less need to seek solutions further afield.

Pharmacological treatments

Although behavioural approaches to intervention are usually the most desirable form of treatment for younger autistic children, there are times when, because of severe behavioural disturbance (especially self-injury or aggression), sleeping problems, overactivity, anxiety or depression, or marked ritualistic and compulsive behaviours, medication may be considered.

However, evaluations of even the most commonly used drugs are frequently inadequate (Lewis 1996). Campbell *et al.* (1996) concluded that only haloperidol, fenfluramine, naltrexone, clomipramine and clonidine have been appropriately investigated, and all of these have their drawbacks and unwanted side-effects. As for the myriad of other pharmacological treatments that have been tried over the years, Campbell *et al.* warn: "No conclusions can be made concerning the efficacy and safety of these agents because the findings are based on small sample sizes and open studies without placebo control." [For updates on the effects of other drug treatments, see recent reviews by Campbell and Cueva (1995), Lewis (1996) and McDougle (1997).]

Educational placement
While there may be no miracle cures for autism, it has long been recognized that the provision of appropriately structured educational programmes is one of the most important aspects of successful treatment (Schopler *et al.* 1971, Rutter and Bartak 1973). Effective teaching programmes (such as TEACCH—Schopler *et al.* 1995) stress the importance of appropriate environmental organization and the use of clear visual cues to circumvent communication difficulties, as well as the need to develop individually based learning programmes. Within this framework, however, there are many different approaches to teaching. The essential component is that educational strategies and curricula should be adapted to the specific patterns of skills and disabilities shown by the child with autism. [For descriptions of a variety of imaginative and innovative techniques that can be used to enhance learning, see Jordan and Powell (1995), Powell and Jordan (1997).] It is also generally more productive—and certainly more rewarding for all concerned—to focus on developing the child's existing skills, rather than attempting to overcome fundamental deficits. Equal emphasis also needs to be placed on meeting children's social and emotional needs.

As noted above, there is good evidence (Rogers 1996) to show that the most effective educational programmes are those that begin early (between the ages of 2 to 4 years). Once the right placement is found this can help greatly to reduce the pressure on families and, if parents, teachers and other professionals work together, this will markedly improve the consistency of management, and ensure the generalization and maintenance of newly acquired behaviours. Thus, good liaison with educational services, to ensure that the child receives early and appropriate provision, is a vital component of any package of care.

Other components of intervention
Finally, it is also important to ensure that the family's needs in other areas are appropriately addressed. Respite care, on a planned and regular basis, can offer parents the rest they often so badly need, provide them with the opportunity to spend time with their other children, and give the child with autism the chance to spend time away from home. Families may also need guidance to ensure that they receive all the benefits to which they are entitled. Money may not improve the child's behaviour but worrying about the lack of it can certainly interfere with parents' ability to cope. Even apparently minor benefits, such as a disabled parking badge, can make the difference between being able to take the child out or not.

The older child with autism may also need help in her/his own right. Cognitive–behavioural strategies to help cope with anxiety, fears or anger may prove effective with older, more able children, although these rarely work in isolation and generally require the cooperation of school and family too. For some children with severe emotional problems, psychoanalytically based interventions may be considered (Maratos 1996), although there is little good evidence that such approaches are helpful (Campbell *et al.* 1996). Nevertheless, for older, more able children with autism, individual psychotherapy or counselling may be useful in helping them to deal with anxiety or depression and the pain that comes from recognizing their difficulties and differences. However, experience suggests that this *must* be combined with direct practical advice on how to deal with problems, otherwise children tend to become preoccupied with the past, or with other possible explanations for their difficulties, making it almost impossible for them to 'move on' in a positive way.

Effective treatment also requires early diagnosis. However, although there is good evidence to show that the most effective intervention programmes are those that begin early—between the ages of 2 to 4 years (Rogers 1996)—diagnosis before the age of 3 years is still rare (Baron-Cohen *et al.* 1996) and the average age for diagnosis (at least in the UK) is around 5.5 years (Howlin and Moore 1997).

Conclusions

Behavioural approaches to the treatment of children with autism have changed almost beyond recognition since they were first introduced over 30 years ago. Interventions are now family and school based, involve naturalistic teaching methods and reward systems, and are designed not according to predetermined programmes but to meet the skills and problems of the individual child as well as the needs of her/his family. The punitive component (including electric shock, noxious tastes or smells, scolding and shouting) of many of the earlier studies has also largely, although not entirely, disappeared. These undoubted improvements, however, have meant that behavioural approaches now require much greater attention to individual and environmental factors than may have been the case in the past. There are no easy recipes, and what works for one child, or for one behaviour, may not be at all effective for others. Careful assessment of individual and family needs is essential before intervention commences, and throughout treatment close monitoring will be required to ensure that intervention procedures maintain their effectiveness, that treatment goals are met, and that the pressure on families is kept to a minimum.

It also seems that the establishment of appropriate management strategies in the early years can help to minimize or even avoid many subsequent behavioural problems (Howlin and Rutter 1987).

First, it is apparent that the development of effective if simple communication strategies from early childhood will almost certainly help to reduce or avoid disruptive behaviours, which may otherwise become the child's principal means of controlling her/his environment (Durand and Carr 1991).

Second, it is essential not to allow or encourage behaviours in young children that will be viewed as 'challenging' or unacceptable as they grow older, not because the behaviour itself has changed, but because other people's perceptions of that behaviour have altered.

Third, behaviours may become unacceptable as individuals become more skilled or determined at carrying them out. An interest in trains may appear innocuous when the child is young; if it later develops into a preoccupation or obsession which is potentially dangerous, as well as being very expensive, the same interest may cause enormous problems.

Fourth, particularly in the case of rituals and obsessions, there is real risk that if such behaviours are not brought under effective control when the child is young, they may steadily escalate until they interfere with many other activities.

Without appropriate help, parents are unlikely to be able to identify potential problems, or will lack the courage and consistency to respond firmly to these, because of fears that resistance will further distress or damage their child. It is the role of professionals to provide families with the information and support they need, in order to enable them to identify problems at an early stage, and to assist them in evolving management strategies that will improve the quality of life for all concerned.

ACKNOWLEDGEMENT

This chapter is based on a paper entitled 'Psychological and educational treatments for autism.' (*Journal of Child Psychology and Psychiatry*, 1998, **39**, 307–322.)

REFERENCES

Attwood, T., Frith U., Hermelin, B. (1988) 'The understanding and use of gestures by autistic and Down's syndrome children.' *Journal of Autism and Developmental Disorders*, **18**, 241–258.

Baron-Cohen, S. (1995) *Mindblindness: an Essay on Autism and Theory of Mind.* Cambridge, MA: MIT Press.

—— Cox, A., Baird, G., Swettenham, J., Nightingale, N., Morgan, K., Drew, A., Charman, T. (1996) 'Psychological markers in the detection of autism in infancy in a large population.' *British Journal of Psychiatry*, **168**, 158–163

Biklen, D. (1993) *Communication Unbound: How Facilitated Communication is Challenging Traditional Views of Autism and Ability/Disability.* New York: Teachers College Press.

Bondy, A., Frost, L. (1996) 'Educational approaches in pre-school: behavior techniques in a public school setting.' *In:* Schopler, E., Mesibov, G.B. (Eds.) *Learning and Cognition in Autism.* New York: Plenum Press, pp. 311–334.

Campbell, M., Cueva, J.E. (1995) 'Psychopharmacology in child and adolescent psychiatry: a review of the past seven years. Part II.' *Journal of the American Academy of Child and Adolescent Psychiatry*, **34**, 1262–1272.

—— Schopler, E., Cueva J.E., Hallin, A. (1996) 'Treatment of autistic disorder.' *Journal of the American Academy of Child and Adolescent Psychiatry*, **35**, 134–143.

Daley, D., Cantrell, R., Cantrell, M., Aman, L. (1972) 'Structuring speech therapy contingencies with an oral apraxic child.' *Journal of Speech and Hearing Disorders*, **37**, 22–32.

Dewart H., Summers, S. (1988) *Pragmatics Profile of Early Communication Skills.* Windsor: NFER.

Dodge K., Schlundt, D., Schocken, I., Delugach, J. (1983) 'Competence and children's sociometric status: the role of peer group entries.' *Merrill-Palmer Quarterly*, **29**, 309–306.

Durand, B.M. (1990) *Severe Behavior Problems: a Functional Communication Approach.* New York: Guilford Press.

—— Carr, E.G. (1991) 'Functional communication training to reduce challenging behaviour: maintenance and application in new settings.' *Journal of Applied Behavior Analysis*, **24**, 251–254.

—— Crimmins, D.B. (1988) 'Identifying the variables maintaining self-injurious behavior.' *Journal of Autism and Developmental Disorders*, **18**, 99–117.

Emerson, E. (1995) *Challenging Behaviour: Analysis and Intervention.* Cambridge: Cambridge University Press.

—— Bromley, J. (1995) 'The form and function of challenging behaviours.' *Journal of Intellectual Disability Research*, **39**, 388–398.

Finnerty, J., Quill, K. (1991) *The Communication Analyzer*. Lexington, MA: Educational Software Research.

Gould, G.A., Rigg, M., Bignell, L. (1991) *The Higashi Experience: the Report of a Visit to the Boston Higashi School*. London: National Autistic Society Publications.

Gunsett, R.P., Mulick, J.A., Fernald W.B., Martin J.L. (1989) 'Brief report: Indications for medical screening prior to behavioral programming for severely and profoundly mentally retarded clients.' *Journal of Autism and Developmental Disorders*, **19**, 167–172

Hadwin, J., Baron-Cohen, S., Howlin, P., Hill, K. (1996) 'Can we teach children with autism to understand emotions, belief or pretence?' *Development and Psychopathology*, **8**, 345–365.

Hall, S. (1997) *The Early Development of Self-Injurious Behaviour in Children with Developmental Disabilities*. PhD thesis, University of London.

Hemsley, R., Howlin, P., Berger, M., Hersov, L., Holbrook, D., Rutter, M., Yule, W. (1978) 'Treating autistic children in a family context.' *In:* Rutter, M, Schopler, E. (Eds.) *Autism: Reappraisal of Concepts and Treatment*. New York: Plenum Press, pp. 379–412.

Hewett, F. (1965) 'Teaching speech to an autistic child through operant conditioning.' *Journal of Orthopsychiatry*, **35**, 927–936.

Hingtgen, J., Trost, F. (1964) 'Shaping cooperative responses in early childhood schizophrenics. III: Reinforcement of mutual physical contact and vocal responses.' *In:* Ulrich, R., Stachnik, T., Mabry, J. (Eds.) *Control of Human Behavior*. Chicago: Scott, Foreman & Co., pp. 136–163.

Howlin, P. (1989) 'Changing approaches to communication training with autistic children.' *British Journal of Disorders of Communication*, **24**, 151–168.

—— (1997a) *Autism: Preparing for Adulthood*. London: Routledge

—— (1997b) 'Prognosis in autism: do specialist treatments affect outcome?' *European Child and Adolescent Psychiatry*, **6**, 55–72.

—— (1998) 'Psychological and educational treatments for autism.' *Journal of Child Psychology and Psychiatry*, **39**, 307–322.

—— Moore, A. (1997) 'Diagnosis in autism: a survey of over 1200 parents.' *Autism: the International Journal of Research and Practice*, **1**, 135–162.

—— Rutter, M. (1987) *Treatment of Autistic Children*. Chichester: Wiley.

—— Yates, P. (1998) 'Increasing social communication skills in young adults with autism attending a social group.' *(In preparation.)*

—— Baron-Cohen, S., Hadwin, J., Swettenham, J. (1998) *Teaching Children with Autism to Mindread. A Practical Manual for Parents and Teachers*. Chichester: Wiley. *(In press.)*

Irlen, H. (1995) 'Viewing the world through rose tinted glasses.' *Communication*, **29** (1), 8–9.

Jolliffe, T., Lansdown, R., Robinson, T. (1992) *Autism: a Personal Account*. London: National Autistic Society.

Jordan, R., Powell, S. (1995) *Understanding and Teaching Children with Autism*. Chichester. Wiley.

Kanner, L. (1973) *Childhood Psychosis: Initial Studies and New Insights*. New York: Winston/Wiley.

Kaufman, B. (1981) *A Miracle to Believe in*. New York: Doubleday.

Kiernan, C. (1983) 'The use of non-vocal communication systems with autistic individuals.' *Journal of Child Psychology and Psychiatry*, **24**, 339–376.

Koegel, R.L., Koegel, L.K. (1995) *Teaching Children with Autism: Strategies for Promoting Positive Interactions and Improving Learning Opportunities*. Baltimore: Paul Brookes.

Konstantareas, M.M. (1987) 'Autistic children exposed to simultaneous communication training.' *Journal of Autism and Developmental Disorders*, **14**, 9–25.

—— Homatidis, S. (1987) 'Ear infections in autistic and normal children.' *Journal of Autism and Developmental Disorders*, **20**, 591–593.

Layton, T.L., Watson, L.R. (1995) 'Enhancing communication in non-verbal children with autism.' *In: Teaching Children with Autism: Strategies to Enhance Communication and Socialization*. New York: Delmar, pp. 73–104.

Lewis, M.H. (1996) 'Brief report: Psychopharmacology of autism spectrum disorders.' *Journal of Autism and Developmental Disorders*, **26**, 231–236.

Lord, C. (1984) 'The development of peer relations in children with autism.' *In:* Morrison, F.J., Lord, C., Keating, D.P. (Eds.) *Applied Developmental Psychology*. New York: Academic Press, pp. 166–230.

—— (1995) 'Facilitating social inclusion: examples from peer intervention programs.' *In:* Schopler, E., Mesibov, G. (Eds.) *Learning and Cognition in Autism*. New York: Plenum Press, pp. 221–239.

—— Rutter, M. (1994) 'Autism and pervasive developmental disorders.' *In:* Rutter, M., Taylor, E., Hersov, L. (Eds.) *Child and Adolescent Psychiatry: Modern Approaches, 3rd Edn*. Oxford: Blackwell, pp. 569–593.

Lovaas, O.I. (1977) *The Autistic Child: Language Development Through Behaviour Modification*. New York: Wiley

—— (1993) 'The development of a treatment—research project for developmentally disabled and autistic children.' *Journal of Applied Behavior Analysis*, **26**, 617–630.

—— (1996) 'The UCLA young autism model of service delivery.' *In:* Maurice, C. (Ed.) *Behavioral Intervention for Young Children with Autism.* Austin, TX: Pro-Ed, pp. 241–250.

—— Berberich, J., Perloff, B., Schaeffer, B. (1966) 'Acquisition of imitative speech in schizophrenic children.' *Science*, **151**, 705–707.

—— Koegel, R., Simmons, J., Stevens, J. (1973) 'Some generalization and follow-up measures on autistic children in behaviour therapy.' *Journal of Applied Behavior Analysis*, **6**, 131–166.

Maratos, O. (1996) 'Psychoanalysis and the management of pervasive developmental disorders, including autism.' *In:* Trevarthen, C., Aitken, K., Papoudi, D., Robarts, J. (Eds.) *Children with Autism: Diagnosis and Interventions to Meet Their Needs.* London: Jessica Kingsley, pp. 161–171.

Marshall, N., Hegrenes, H. (1972) 'The use of the written word as a communication system for non-verbal autistic children.' *Journal of Speech and Hearing Disorders*, **39**, 186–194.

McDougle, C.J. (1997) 'Psychopharmacology.' *In:* Cohen, D., Volkmar, F. (Eds.) *Handbook of Autism and Pervasive Developmental Disorders, 2nd Edn.* New York: Wiley, pp. 707–729.

—— Naylor, S.T., Cohen, D.J., Volkmar, F.R., Heninger, G.R., Price, L.H. (1996) 'A double blind, placebo-controlled study of fluvoxamine in adults with autistic disorder.' *Archives of General Psychiatry*, **53**, 1001–1008.

McEachin, J.J., Smith, T., Lovaas, O.I. (1993) 'Long-term outcome for children with autism who received early intensive behavioral treatment.' *American Journal of Mental Retardation*, **97**, 359–372.

Mesibov, G.B. (1984) 'Social skills training with verbal autistic adolescents and adults: a program model.' *Journal of Autism and Developmental Disorders*, **14**, 395–404.

—— (1993) 'Treatment outcome is encouraging: comments on McEachin *et al.*' *American Journal of Mental Retardation*, **97**, 379–380.

Oliver, C. (1995) 'Self injurious behaviour in children with learning disabilities: recent advances in assessment and intervention.' *Journal of Child Psychology and Psychiatry*, **36**, 909–928.

Owens, R.G., MacKinnon, S. (1993) 'The functional analysis of challenging behaviours: some conceptual and theoretical problems.' *In:* Jones, R.S.P., Eayrs, C.B. (Eds.) *Challenging Behaviour and Intellectual Disability: a Psychological Perspective.* Avon: BILD Publications, pp. 224–239.

Ozonoff, S., Miller, J. (1995) 'Teaching Theory of Mind: a new approach to social skills training for individuals with autism.' *Journal of Autism and Developmental Disorders*, **25**, 415–434.

Perry, R., Cohen, I., DeCarlo, R. (1995) 'Case study: deterioration, autism and recovery in two siblings.' *Journal of the American Academy of Child and Adolescent Psychiatry*, **34**, 233–237.

Powell, S., Jordan, R. (Eds.) (1997) *Autism and Learning: a Guide to Good Practice*. London. David Fulton.

Prizant, B., Schuler, A. (1987) 'Facilitating communication: language approaches.' *In:* Cohen, D., Donnellan, A. (Eds.) *Handbook of Autism and Pervasive Developmental Disorders.* New York: Wiley, pp. 316–332.

—— —— Wetherby, A., Rydell, P. (1997) 'Enhancing language and communication development: language approaches.' *In:* Cohen, D., Volkmar, F. (Eds.) *Handbook of Autism and Pervasive Developmental Disorders, 2nd Edn.* New York: Wiley, pp. 572–605.

Quill, K.A. (1995) *Teaching Children with Autism: Strategies to Enhance Communication and Socialization.* New York: Delmar.

Richer, J., Zappella, M. (1989) 'Changing social behaviour: the place of Holding.' *Communication*, **23** (2), 35–39.

Rimland, B., Edelson, S.M. (1994) 'The effects of Auditory Integration Training on autism.' *American Journal of Speech–Language Pathology*, **5**, 16–24.

—— —— (1995) 'Brief report: A pilot study of Auditory Integration Training in autism.' *Journal of Autism and Developmental Disorders*, **25**, 61–70

Roeyers, H. (1996) 'The influence of nonhandicapped peers on the social interaction of children with a pervasive developmental disorder.' *Journal of Autism and Developmental Disorders*, **26**, 303–320.

Rogers, S.J. (1996) 'Brief report: early intervention in autism.' *Journal of Autism and Developmental Disorders*, **26**, 243–246.

Rinaldi, W. (1992) *The Social Use of Language Programme.* Oxford, NFER–Nelson.

Risley, T., Wolf, M. (1967) 'Establishing functional speech in echolalic children.' *Behaviour Research and Therapy*, **5**, 73–88.

Rutter, M. (1996) 'Autism research: prospects and priorities.' *Journal of Autism and Developmental Disorders*, **26**, 257–276.

—— (1985) 'Infantile autism and other pervasive developmental disorders.' *In:* Rutter, M., Hersov, L. (Eds.) *Child and Adolescent Psychiatry: Modern Approaches, 2nd Edn.* Oxford: Blackwell, pp. 545–566.

—— Bartak, L. (1973) 'Special educational treatment of autistic children: a comparative study. II. Follow-up findings and implications for services.' *Journal of Child Psychology and Psychiatry*, **14**, 241–270.

Rydell, P.J., Mirenda P. (1994) 'The effects of high and low constraint utterances on the production of immediate and delayed echolalia in young children with autism.' *Journal of Autism and Developmental Disorders*, **24**, 719–730.

—— Prizant, B. (1995) 'Assessment and intervention strategies for children who use echolalia.' *In:* Quill, K.A. (Ed.) *Teaching Children with Autism: Strategies to Enhance Communication and Socialization.* New York: Delmar, pp. 105–132.

Schopler, E., Reichler, R.J. (1971) 'Parents as co-therapists in the treatment of psychotic children.' *Journal of Autism and Childhood Schizophrenia*, **1**, 87–102.

—— Brehm, S.S., Kinsbourne, M., Reichler, R.J. (1971) 'Effects of treatment structure on development in autistic children.' *Archives of General Psychiatry*, **20**, 174–181.

—— Short, A., Mesibov, G. (1989) 'Relation of behavioral treatment to "normal functioning": comment on Lovaas.' *Journal of Consulting and Clinical Psychology*, **57**, 162–164.

—— Mesibov, G.B., Hearsey, K. (1995) 'Structured teaching in the TEACCH system.' *In:* Schopler, E., Mesibov G.B. (Eds.) *Learning and Cognition in Autism.* New York: Plenum Press, pp. 243–267.

Schuler, A.L., Peck, C.A., Willard, C., Theimer, K. (1989) 'Assessment of communicative means and functions through interview: assessing the communicative capabilities of individuals with limited language.' *Seminars in Speech and Language*, **10**, 51–61.

—— Prizant, B., Wetherby, A. (1997) 'Enhancing language and communication development: prelinguistic approaches.' *In:* Cohen, D., Volkmar, F. (Eds.) *Handbook of Autism and Pervasive Developmental Disorders, 2nd Edn.* New York: Wiley, pp. 539–571.

Short, A. (1984) 'Short term treatment outcome using parents as therapists for their own children.' *Journal of Child Psychology and Psychiatry*, **25**, 443–458.

Stehli, A. (1992) *The Sound of a Miracle: A Child's Triumph Over Autism.* New York: Doubleday.

Sturmey, P. (1995) 'Analog baselines: a critical review of the methodology.' *Research in Developmental Disabilities*, **16**, 269–284.

—— (1996) *Functional Analysis in Clinical Psychology.* Chichester: Wiley.

Swettenham, J. (1996) 'Can children with autism be taught to understand false beliefs using computers?' *Journal of Child Psychology and Psychiatry*, **37**, 157–165.

Trevarthen, C., Aitken, K., Papoudi, D., Roberts, J.M. (1996) *Children with Autism. Diagnosis and Interventions to Meet Their Needs.* London: Jessica Kingsley.

Walker, M. (1980) *The Makaton Vocabulary. Revised Edition.* Camberley, Surrey: Makaton Vocabulary Development Project.

Welch, M. (1988) *Holding Time.* London: Century Hutchinson.

Wetherby, A., Schuler, A., Prizant, B. (1997) 'Enhancing language and communication development: theoretical foundations.' *In:* Cohen, D., Volkmar, F. (Eds) *Handbook of Autism and Pervasive Developmental Disorders, 2nd Edn.* New York: Wiley, pp. 513–538.

Williams, T.I. (1989) 'A social skills group for autistic children.' *Journal of Autism and Developmental Disorders*, **19**, 143–156.

Wolf, M., Risley, T., Mees, H. (1964) 'Applications of operant conditioning procedures to the behaviour problems of an autistic child.' *Behaviour Research and Therapy*, **1**, 305–312.

Wolfberg, P.J., Schuler, A.L. (1993) 'Integrated play groups: a model for promoting the social and cognitive dimensions of play.' *Journal of Autism and Developmental Disorders*, **23**, 1–23.

Yoder, P., Layton, T. (1988) 'Speech following sign language training in autistic children with minimal verbal language.' *Journal of Autism and Developmental Disorders*, **18**, 217–230.

4
CHILDREN WITH LEARNING DISABILITIES

Janet Carr

Children with learning disabilities, by definition, have special problems in acquiring the skills they need in life. They learn more slowly, and may be less able to learn from ordinary teaching methods. Some of the methods used most commonly with normally developing children—talk, discussion, explanation—may not be so appropriate if the child has limited understanding of speech. Similarly the threat of sanctions—"If you do that again I'll stop your pocket money for a week"—may not mean much to a child who cannot easily imagine the future. However, just like other children they need to learn skills and ways of behaving that will help them to function in and be welcomed by society, and ways to help them to achieve this must be sought.

Four important ways of working towards this aim will be addressed in this chapter: (i) looking at the behaviour; (ii) encouraging appropriate or desirable behaviours; (iii) teaching such behaviours; (iv) managing inappropriate or undesirable behaviours.

Looking at behaviours

Before starting to do anything about a behaviour, it may be useful to spend some time just observing it. This may seem like a waste of time—why not get on with dealing with it? While sympathizing with this point of view, a short time spent in observation really does help. It enables the observer to:

- be clear about what is going on;
- decide exactly what, at the outset, to try to do;
- get a good picture of the here-and-now, which later can be compared with the results of any remedial programme.

Having decided on the target behaviour (*e.g.* Mary cannot dress herself, Tom screams a lot), a period of time is set (usually about a week) over which the behaviour will be watched and recorded. During this time no new strategy to deal with it will be attempted—it will simply be handled as it was before. If the behaviour is one that crops up only occasionally it can be noted every time it occurs. If it happens a great deal this every-time approach may be too much to cope with, and one or two times in the day may then be chosen in which to make observations, *e.g.* 10–11 a.m., or if energy permits, perhaps 5–6 p.m. as well. The actual times are not important, but if possible times should be chosen when the behaviour is most likely to happen; these times should then be kept to.

A useful extra, again if energy permits, is to note not only the behaviour but two other things as well: first, what was going on just before the behaviour happened—who else was around? was the child happy/tired/unwell/hungry?—and second, what happened next—how did those around respond? and how did the child react to that? This ABC (Antecedents, Behaviour and Consequences) approach, although more laborious, can provide information that will help decide how to go about tackling the problem. It is, however, a good deal more complex than simply keeping a count of the behaviours, which in itself can provide a great deal of information.

Earlier it was said that a note would be made of the occurrence of the behaviour: that is, a written record. Observations that are written down at the time are much more useful than those stored only in the memory. It is easier to keep written records if a record sheet has already been made out, preferably in such a way that just a tick has to be put in a column rather than requiring a lot of writing to be done each time. For example, Timmy's problem was temper tantrums; his mother kept a sheet of paper pinned up on the kitchen wall, with the days of the week running down the side. Each time he had a tantrum she put a tick on the line for that day. If she had been doing an ABC-type record she might also have had spaces for the time of day, who else was around at the time, or any other information she thought would help, like this:

Timmy's tantrums

Day	Time	People	Antecedents: Tired (T), Bored (B), Unwell (U), Hungry (H), Other (O)	Consequences
Mon 12	5.05	Ann, me	T, O – came home from school upset	I tried to calm him by stroking, no effect. Tantrum stopped after 10 minutes.

Another way of observing and recording observations is to use Momentary Time Sampling (MTS). Here, instead of the behaviour being recorded every time it happens, it is recorded only at certain times. Lucy used to suck brushes, any brushes, up to and including the lavatory brush, and her mother wanted to teach her not to do this. She chose 4–6 p.m. as her observation time, but because that was a busy time for her she decided to use MTS. She divided the time into quarter hour periods (4–4.15, 4.15–4.30 and so on), and in the last half minute of each period she went to check on Lucy. If at that time she was sucking a brush, her mother put a tick on the chart; if she was not, she put a cross. As the name indicates, this method 'samples' the behaviour, and may not catch every instance of it, but provided the times decided on are kept to—Lucy's mother was careful not to record brush-sucking in between times just because she happened to notice it—it is a good method, and better for busy people than not taking records at all.

This record of observations taken before the problem is tackled (known as a baseline) can have some useful spin-offs. It is quite common to find that, when it is painstakingly recorded, the behaviour is not as bad as had been thought. Ann's problem was disobedience ("she won't do a thing I ask her"). For her baseline her mother elected to record how often Ann did as she was asked—"there won't be anything on the chart". The observations done, Ann's mother brought her chart back with some surprise: "There *are* some ticks." Occasionally too there may the bonus of the behaviour fading away over the course of the observations. Lucy's mother found her sucking brushes less and less during the 4–6 p.m. time until she was not doing it at all. "But she's doing it just as much at other times" said her mother, so those other times also had to be tackled. Nevertheless it was a great thrill for her to see that this undesirable behaviour could be reduced in so simple a way.

Encouraging behaviours

Everyone needs encouragement. Children with learning disabilities perhaps need it more than most, and are more likely than most to miss out on it. In order to help them learn they may need to be deliberately rewarded, or reinforced, when they show the desired behaviours. (Although 'reward' is a more familiar term, 'reinforcement' will be used in this chapter because its meaning is slightly different and it is a more appropriate term in this context.)

Reinforcement is defined as anything which, when it follows a behaviour, makes that behaviour more likely to happen again. Note that this does not necessarily imply 'something nice'. Reinforcement is *anything* that makes the behaviour more likely to happen again. This means that the child must be studied (observed) carefully (or known very well) to determine what in her/his case can be expected to be reinforcing. Then the reinforcer is tried out, to see whether its use does lead to an increase in the behaviour. Many of the things that are reinforcing for children with learning disabilities *are* things that are generally considered pleasant—a sweet, music, praise, approval. However, some things that are thought of as pleasant, such as praise, for some children have no effect on their behaviour; and some of the things that are reinforcing for some children are not, for most of us, pleasant at all. One child, for example, liked to lick a bar of soap, another to suck ice cubes. Thus no assumptions are made about what things will be reinforcing for any particular child; for those not already very familiar with the child, they must be discovered through observation.

TYPES OF REINFORCERS

There are a number of different kinds of reinforcers. Foods and drinks are obvious examples, not just sweets but also fruit, nuts, cheese, sultanas, fruit juice, cola, lemonade, tea, coffee, or sometimes just plain water. Then there are all the ways of showing approval—hugs, kisses, praise, cuddles. Music, bright lights, and other sounds and sensations are much enjoyed by some children, though they may be very specific in what they will respond to: one child would only respond to extracts from a particular Peter Rabbit record, another only to Tommy Dorsey records. Toys and games, outings, treats and privileges like going swimming or being taken to a football match can also work well, though many of these are too significant (or expensive) to be given for individual instances of behaviour: their use is discussed under 'Star Charts and Token Programmes' (below).

Sometimes, for a particular child, it can be difficult to find anything that works. Then an approach can be adopted called the Premack Principle (after the American psychologist David Premack). The Principle states: 'A high-frequency behaviour may be used to reinforce a low-frequency behaviour.' According to this, anything the child does when left to her/his own devices may be used as a reinforcer for that child. Thus, if when left alone the child rocks, or, in the case of Timmy, twiddles a small plastic cup on the tip of his thumb, it may be possible to teach more useful things by allowing rocking or twiddling only when he has done the required task. This may sound odd, and some parents worry that by following such

80

a procedure they may actually encourage the stereotyped behaviour. However, the Principle has often been used very successfully. Becky, whose preferred activity was to run full tilt round the room, was allowed to do so only when she had sat still for a few seconds. Gradually the time for which she had to sit was lengthened until eventually she would sit for a meal or a lesson before having her run.

HOW AND WHEN TO GIVE REINFORCEMENT

When working with a child with learning disabilities it seems particularly important that the reinforcement be given immediately after the behaviour. Delay makes the connection between the behaviour and the reinforcer less clear. There is also the risk that it will allow some other behaviour—e.g. hand-flapping or tooth-grinding—to occur between the behaviour and the arrival of the reinforcement, so that in effect what would be reinforced would be the flapping or grinding. It has been found that even a delay as short as five seconds can slow down learning. So the reinforcer needs to be immediately at hand, to be given to the child as soon as the behaviour occurs.

As far as possible, the reinforcer should not be given at other times. For instance, if the reinforcer is a special biscuit it will help if the child does not also get it at teatime. If praise or attention is the reinforcer then of course the child will be given it at other times, but the warmest enthusiasm is reserved for any occurrence of the appropriate behaviour.

STAR CHARTS AND TOKEN PROGRAMMES

Many people will be familiar with the idea of star charts. They have often been used, for example, to help children (including children with learning disabilities) to become toilet trained—every day with dry pants or every night with a dry bed leads to a star being stuck on a chart. This is fine as far as it goes, and if it works. Children with learning disabilities are not always motivated by the charts that work with normally developing children, but with a bit of adjustment they can be very effective. Thus, a system is set up whereby the stars, instead of being all the child gets for her/his good behaviour, are exchangeable for things s/he wants. Each instance of behaviour earns a star, and a certain number of stars have to be earned before they can be exchanged. Then all sorts of larger things—the treats and privileges mentioned above—become available for exchange. At the same time, because the child knows that the stars will lead to something s/he wants—the 'back-up reinforcer'—the stars themselves become reinforcing and the child will make an effort for them.

Ann's mother wanted to help Ann to be less disobedient, so she decided to give her a star every time she did as she was asked. Her mother knew that Ann very much wanted a particular CD: as this was quite expensive she decided that Ann would have to earn 60 stars for it. Although this sounds a daunting number, Ann was so thrilled at the thought of getting the CD she threw herself into the task. Not only did she do as she was asked on a great many more occasions than had previously been the case but she often now offered to help her mother.

In setting up a programme like this four things need to be done. First, the behaviour that needs to change must be identified. If it is a skill to be learned, a star can be given for every time the child does it (or some part of it, see 'Teaching Methods' below). If it is a problem behaviour this may be tackled, as Ann's mother did, by reinforcing its opposite—Ann, who was disobedient, was reinforced for obedience—or a star may be given for periods of time when the behaviour does not occur. Leroy used to lash out randomly at people, so he was given a star for each half hour in which he had not hit anyone.

Second, it must be decided how many stars will be given. At the beginning this is quite simple; one star is given for each instance or period of the desired behaviour. Later the child may need to do more for the stars—this is discussed under 'Adapting the programme' (see below).

Next come two things that are closely connected, the back-up reinforcer and the number of stars needed to earn it. The back-up reinforcer will be, as always, something the child very much wants. It may be something quite small, like a can of cola or five minutes with a tape recorder, or something as significant as a meal out or a trip to the zoo or to a football match. When one of these major items is seen as a good reinforcer for the child it is important to make sure that it really can be delivered: is it affordable? and, if it is something that requires another person, for example to take the child out, will there definitely be someone available to do this when the trip has been earned? Chaos will ensue if the situation arises where the child earns all the stars and then cannot get the chosen reinforcer. How many stars are needed for the reinforcer depends partly on how significant the reinforcer is: major things cannot be given too often, so a large number of stars may be needed for them, like the 60 that Ann had to get for her CD. This also means that, if a child finds it difficult to wait a long time for the reinforcer, a smaller one that can be obtained more quickly should be decided upon. It may be especially important to do this at first, when the child needs to find that the system does work and that if s/he does what is asked the reinforcer really will be forthcoming. Later, if there are larger things s/he wants, s/he may by that time be better able to wait for them. In fact it can be a good strategy to have a varied 'menu' of reinforcers to draw on—an iced lolly, an outing to the park, a glass of orange juice, staying up late to watch a video—so that each time a new programme is set up the child can choose which it should be this time: whether s/he will aim to get a minor reinforcer quickly or opt for a grander target over a longer period of time will be up to her/him.

ADAPTING THE PROGRAMME

In the early stages of an intervention, the programme is set up on the basis of the best information available about the child's behaviour and what is likely to be an effective reinforcer for her/him. This usually involves a good bit of guesswork, so it can happen that, as time goes on, changes are needed. Often this will mean changing the number of stars the child gets or the number s/he has to exchange for the reinforcer. If rather too high a standard has been set, so that the child is struggling to amass enough stars (perhaps getting a bit discouraged), either the number of stars s/he gets can be increased, or the number s/he needs to give can be reduced. Alternatively, sights may have been set too low, or the child gets better at the task and is earning stars extremely rapidly. Of course this is what was hoped for; it shows that the child is eager to get the reinforcers and that s/he can do the task well enough to get them. But if s/he can get them so freely, enough may not be being asked of her/him, while s/he may also quickly get tired of the reinforcer. In this case the number of stars s/he gets may be reduced, or the 'price' of the reinforcer may be increased slightly; the latter often seems easier and better in practice.

When it is realized that changes are necessary they will not usually be made in mid-programme: ideally, the current chart should be completed and the reinforcer given, and then a new chart drawn up with spaces for more or fewer stars (depending on whether the child has been getting the stars too quickly or not quickly enough). If a new reinforcer is to be introduced this is an opportunity to negotiate a new 'price level'. When Ann had earned her 60 stars and got her CD, she wanted to work next for a pair of pretty knickers; although these were actually cheaper than the CD her mother said she would need 80 stars for them. By now Ann was so obliging that she earned the knickers in little more than the time it had taken her to get the CD.

FINING

A system that involves giving stars leads some people to the idea that stars could also be taken away for undesirable behaviour: that they could be used in punishment programmes. I have never been very successful in using stars in this way, and am not keen on it. However, there is a variant of this approach, first described by Salend and Kovalich (1981), which I have found useful and which I call 'free-star fining'. Whereas when ordinary fining is used, the stars that are taken away have already been earned, in free-star fining a number of stars are *given* to the child at the outset; then any occurrence of the inappropriate behaviour results in the removal of one of these free stars. If at the end of the period decided on there are any stars left, the child is entitled to the full amount of reinforcement.

Like stimulus control (see below), this approach means accepting that some unwanted behaviour will occur, so it is not an appropriate method to use for the most serious or dangerous behaviours. Ted's verbal abuse of staff and other children in his school, although not dangerous, was bad enough for him to be threatened with suspension, and a 'free-star fining' programme was set up for him. At the beginning of each day he was given 15 stickers, put up on a wall at ceiling level (out of reach for him and for other children). Any 10-second bout of abuse led to a staff member removing one of the stickers. At the end of the day if any sticker remained Ted was entitled to his chosen reinforcer. Subsequently it is planned gradually to reduce the number of stickers Ted is given each day, so that fewer and fewer episodes of abuse will become acceptable. Simultaneously Ted is to be given (separate) reinforcement for any pleasant remark he makes to any child or member of staff.

This programme has only just started so it is not possible to report on its outcome. However, that by Salend and Kovalich, on a whole classful of disruptive children, was highly successful.

ENDING PROGRAMMES

The programmes described are intended to help a child to get over a particular problem: they are not meant to go on for ever. Nevertheless, it is important not to end a programme abruptly. Instead they need to be planned to fade out gradually. So, once the child can perform the task easily, instead of the reinforcer being given for every occurrence of 'good' behaviour it is given every second or third, then every fourth or fifth time. Still better, instead of keeping to a rigid schedule the times of delivery will be varied; thus, the reinforcer might be given after the behaviour has occurred once, then twice, then twice again, then once, then three times, then twice. Counting up, there were 11 occurrences of the behaviour and the reinforcer was given six times. This means that *on average* the reinforcer was given about every second time, although the times it was actually given were varied. Later, if the child is still doing well, the reinforcement schedule may be 'thinned' still further so that the child is rewarded on average every third or fourth time. The good thing about this 'variable' schedule is that, as the child gets the reinforcer irregularly, s/he does not expect it at any particular time. So if it does not appear at any one time s/he does not get upset and give up hope of it, but carries on working for it. In technical jargon this is called 'resistance to extinction', and is a bonus when the behaviour is a desirable one. (It is a very different matter when the behaviour is an undesirable one, and this will be discussed later.)

Few people outside psychological laboratories are going to work out and stick to such elaborate schedules but it is quite possible to be more informal, giving the reinforcer from time to time but not at regular intervals. In this case it is a good idea, especially at first, not to leave too long gaps between reinforcers, so occasionally the reinforcer may be given after only one occurrence of the behaviour.

Although a plan should usually be made for fading the reinforcers once the behaviour is well established, it may not always be necessary to do this. Occasionally the programme just quietly peters out, and the child keeps up the good behaviour without needing the stars or reinforcers. Philip's family used a very successful programme to teach him to sleep in his own bed, rather than climb into his parents' bed as he had done almost every night for most of the four and a half years of his life. After a few weeks he seemed to lose interest in the stars and the reinforcer but continued to sleep in his own bed—perhaps it was just that a habit had been broken. Sometimes other more natural reinforcers take over: the child finds s/he enjoys the learned activity for its own sake; or the praise and attention people give are pleasurable; or the behaviour may eventually become second nature. Tom went through all these stages. A quite elaborate programme, using food reinforcers, was used to teach him to dress himself. Once he could do this well he went on dressing himself, at first because he was so proud of his new skill and showed it off every day to his admiring family. Later he simply dressed himself as everyone does, as the normal start to the day.

Teaching methods

In the previous section ways were discussed of encouraging the child to carry out appropriate or desirable behaviours, by reinforcing them when they occur. However, if children need to learn a *new* skill, encouragement, on its own, may not be enough: instead they may need to learn what it is that they are to do. For children with learning disabilities the usual ways of teaching—telling, describing, explaining, even showing—do not always work, and other methods may be needed. This section is concerned with some of these other teaching methods: shaping; prompts; breaking the activity down into small steps; and chaining.

SHAPING

When shaping is used the first thing to do is to explore how much of the skill the child can already do, and start by reinforcing her/him for doing that much; then the reinforcer is kept back until s/he (perhaps accidentally) does a tiny bit more, then a tiny bit more still, and so on. Simon was 11 years old and refused to clean his teeth or allow them to be cleaned. He was quite happy to go into the bathroom and wander about it but would not go near the washbasin. So at first he was reinforced if his wanderings took him within a metre of the washbasin. Soon he was quite comfortable with that. Then he was reinforced if he went within 60 cm of the washbasin, then 30 cm. Next he was reinforced if he came within 30 cm of the washbasin when a toothbrush was lying on it, then if he touched the toothbrush; and so on.

Shaping is a slow method and relies on children making the 'next step' action of their own accord in order for that to be reinforced. Other methods are in many cases quicker and more effective. Nevertheless, shaping is sometimes the only possible method to use (for example if the child very much dislikes being touched), while the idea that it can be useful to reinforce a child for a behaviour that is not precisely the one wanted is worth bearing in mind.

PROMPTS

Prompts are ways of helping the child to do the required behaviours. There are three main kinds: physical, gestural and verbal, as well as environmental or structural prompts which can also be very helpful.

When physical prompts are used the child is guided—the hands, feet, head and in some cases the whole body are moved—to carry out the task s/he needs to learn. At the start the child may be initiating little of the action, but s/he feels her/his limbs and body doing it; and because s/he is reinforced for the completed action s/he is more ready to try to do it next time.

Darren could feed himself quite well but could not cut up his food, and his mother wanted to teach him this. He was very fond of chips so she made some and put them on his plate. Darren sat on his chair and picked up his knife in his right hand and his fork in his left hand. His mother stood behind his chair, and put her hands over his, right over right and left over left. She moved his left hand to impale a chip with his fork. She said, "Cut the chip, Darren." With her right hand over his right hand she made him cut the chip. When it was in half she said "Well done, Darren!" and let him put the piece of chip in his mouth, and then made him lower the knife and fork to the plate. When he had eaten both halves of the first chip they did the same thing with another.

At this point, although Darren was holding the knife it was his mother who was making all the back and forth sawing movements. Darren, however, was learning what this felt like, and after a time his mother began to sense that he was doing some of it. She then lessened her efforts, letting Darren do as much as he could. Later she was able to do still less, until Darren was doing all the sawing, although for a time after this she kept her hands just above his ('shadowing' his hands) ready to help if he needed it. This process, where the prompter gradually leaves off the action as the child takes it over, is known as 'fading'. It is very important and perhaps not as easy as it sounds. Judgements (sometimes mistaken) have constantly to be made as to how much the child can do and how much help is still required. The child should always do as much as s/he can, but should not be allowed to go too fast and fail.

Gestural prompts are those movements, often made during speech, which also convey meaning: "Jim, go over there, by that tree"—pointing to the tree. Gestures can help a child to know what is meant. For instance, you say "Sit down" and point to the chair: the child may or may not know what "Sit down" means but the pointing finger makes it more likely that s/he will understand what is wanted. Gestures can be quite powerful in helping children with learning disabilities to understand, and not just large arm movements: a jerk of the head or even a glance can give the message. One may say, "Give me the book, Julie" and glance at the book; Julie may not know what the word 'book' means but she sees the glance go to the object on the table and she hands over the book. This can lead to people thinking she can understand more than she really does (and perhaps getting annoyed with her if she does not always respond as they expect), especially as such a tiny gesture may be made quite unconsciously.

Verbal prompts tell the child in words what to do, and if s/he understands the words they help her/him to know what is needed. Verbal prompts are the ones most people use and are accustomed to responding to—"If you're going to the supermarket, can you get a dozen eggs and some biscuits?". Children with learning disabilities often have difficulty with words. If they cannot understand the words, then, however willing they may be, they cannot carry out the instructions that flow so naturally from the adults around them. In that case physical prompting, linked perhaps with some simple verbal prompts, may make it easier for them to respond.

Like physical prompts, gestural and verbal prompts can be faded, and indeed should be if the child is eventually to be independent of them. Gestural prompts become shorter and weaker, a jerk of the head becoming just a twitch; a verbal prompt can become shorter—'Say hello' goes to 'Say hel..', then even fainter until it is just a whisper.

Changes in the surroundings, or structural prompts, are another way to help the child to learn. Instead of asking them to do something different, something around them is changed which makes it easier for them to learn. Thus, learning to put on a jumper may begin with one that is loose, especially round the neck. A child learning to self-feed may do better with cutlery whose handles have been enlarged (Plastozote* is good for this) and with a non-slip mat under the plate to steady it. Extra-large buttons and buttonholes will help a child who is beginning to learn to fasten shirts. Drinking was a problem for Timmy: he would not drink out of a cup but would only take sips out of a spoon. He eventually learnt to drink out of a cup by being given his drinks out of a series of spoons that gradually, over a total of eight months, became deeper, and the handle more curved, until it bent over to touch the side of the 'spoon'. By now it was indistinguishable from a cup, and after this Timmy drank out of cups like everyone else.

Structural prompts make it easier for the children to learn. Like other prompts, as the child becomes more skilful the prompts are, wherever possible, faded so that in the end s/he can put on any jumper, use ordinary cutlery and crockery and button up any garment.

*Plastozote tubing obtainable from: Nottingham Rehab Ltd, 17 Ludlow Hill Road, West Bridgford, Nottinghamshire, NG2 6HD.

BREAKING THE ACTIVITY DOWN INTO SMALL STEPS (TASK ANALYSIS)
Many of the skills a child needs to learn are too complex to tackle all at once. Jack needed to learn to dress himself, but that was far too much for him to attempt so a start was made with his vest. However, even that was too much, so putting on a vest was broken down into a series of smaller steps, as: (1) pick up vest; (2) pull vest over head; (3) put one arm through armhole; (4) put other arm through armhole; (5) pull vest down.

These steps may still be too big, and some may need to be broken down further. For example, step 2 might become: (2a) pull halfway over head; (2b) pull right over head. Steps 3 and 4 might become: (3/4a) double up arm under vest, with hand almost to armhole; (3/4b) push arm through armhole.

How small the steps need to be depends on what the child can cope with, but a good general rule is to make them smaller rather than bigger. If they are too small, all that happens is that the child goes through them quickly. If a step is too big s/he may not be able to manage it at all.

CHAINING
Once a scale has been drawn up for the skill the child needs to learn, s/he can be taught first one step, then the next; then these two steps can be joined together, or *chained*, so that s/he then does them almost as one action. Which end of the process to start at has also to be decided . Starting at the beginning (*i.e.* with step 1, pick up vest) seems the most natural, and is called *forward chaining*. Often, however, *backward chaining* is preferred, which involves teaching the last step in the chain first. This may sound an odd way to go about it, but it means that, with the child mastering the last step, reinforcement follows straight away. When Jack was being taught to put on his vest his teacher began by carrying out all the first four steps. Then she prompted Jack to pull the vest down: she put his hands on the bottom edge of the vest and, with her hands over his, helped him to pull it down. The task was completed and at once Jack got his reinforcement. When he was able to do step 5 quite by himself she moved on to step 4, prompting him to put the second arm through the armhole, later fading the prompt for this too. Then she went on to step 3, and so on.

Using these techniques, and especially physical prompts and task analysis, children with learning difficulties can successfully learn tasks that may at first have seemed quite beyond them.

Managing undesirable/inappropriate behaviours
So far this chapter has been mostly about teaching children new skills, and this will always be the most important focus for those with learning difficulties. Like other children, however, they will from time to time do undesirable things, and will need help to get rid of these behaviours. This is not only because the behaviours are inconvenient or unpleasant for other people: they may also have unpleasant consequences for the children themselves, ranging from damaging their chances of learning to self-injury. John's rocking took up so much of his time that he could not be taught to play, and Carol's eye-poking was reducing further what sight she had. These behaviours had to be tackled for the children's sakes.

The ways in which these inappropriate behaviours were tackled may seem a bit unusual.

For most children, when they misbehave, punishment follows—either a scolding, or some penalty, like the forfeiture of pocket money. Punishment is meant both to teach the children to behave better in the future and, in at least a small way, to make them suffer for what they have done. Where children with learning disabilities are concerned, there is no interest in making them suffer. They should be helped to have the most enjoyable lives possible, and this may include their learning *not* to do some things. The methods used are those which, when they follow a behaviour, *make that behaviour less likely to happen again*. This is the opposite of the definition of reinforcement given above. Similarly it does not imply that what will follow the behaviour will be something unpleasant. In fact some of the things that might be thought of as undesirable, like a severe telling-off, may not reduce the behaviour at all, while something very mild, like looking away from the child for a few moments, may do so. As with reinforcement, the question to ask is: what effect does the method have on the behaviour of that particular child?

There are a couple of preliminary things that can be done.

UNDERSTANDING THE BEHAVIOUR

As already emphasized, before tackling an undesirable behaviour some time should be spent observing it. It is important to establish exactly what it is, when and where it is most likely to happen, how people react to it, and so on. In doing so answers to another question may emerge—What is the point of this behaviour and what is the child getting out of it? In particular it may become apparent, especially for a child who cannot communicate easily, that the behaviour is the child's way of trying to convey a message. Alan used to give high-pitched screams when he was taken to shops or the supermarket; eventually it was realized that he was distressed by the noise of these places, and was trying to say "I can't stand all this racket." He was not deliberately trying to be annoying but he could not tell people how he felt; all he could do was scream. Once the message behind the scream was understood, a way of helping him could be found. In other cases children may have tantrums, or throw things, or lash out. If observation shows that they do these things when they want or don't want something, it may be possible to teach them a more acceptable way of making their wants known. Perhaps the first thing to try would be to teach the child to make a sign for what s/he wants. Some children will already do this, making signs that people can recognize. For example, Edmund used to clutch the front of his trousers when he wanted to go to the toilet. This was quite effective, but he got some funny looks when he was out in public so he was taught the Makaton* sign for 'toilet'. Besides being more discreet, Makaton signs are quite widely known so there was a good chance that people would understand what he wanted. If signing is too difficult for a child s/he can be given pictures of the things s/he most often wants, which s/he can point to when s/he needs them. Derek used to have a chain necklace (the sort used for identity photographs) with pictures of a drink, the toilet, his bed, and so on, so that he could pick out and point to the one he wanted at that moment. The pictures gave him a way of letting people know at least some of his wants without him throwing a tantrum.

*Makaton Vocabulary Development Project, 31 Firwood Drive, Camberley, Surrey, GU15 3QD.

When the child is first taught an alternative way of expressing her/his needs, the reinforcer will be being given what s/he has asked for. However, in time it may not always be possible for the child to have what s/he wants, and this may sometimes have to be refused. Nevertheless s/he can be shown that the request has been understood, even if it cannot immediately be complied with. David, who could not talk, used to hit people, apparently for no reason. He very much liked going out for walks, and it became clear that he hit people most often when he wanted to go out. He was taught the sign for 'Out', and at first every time he made the sign he was taken out. Later he could not be taken out so often. His teacher told him that she understood that he wanted to go out, that unfortunately he could not be taken out right away, but that he would be taken out as soon as possible. David came to realize that he had been understood, and, although he did not much like it, he could wait; and he *was* taken out as soon as this could be done.

TAKING AVOIDING ACTION
One of the simple ways to deal with a problem behaviour is to prevent or avoid it by altering things in the child's surroundings that will make the behaviour less likely to occur. This strategy is used in many ordinary households with small children: rather than spending a lot of time preventing them from doing harm, bleach and medicines are stored out of their way, and delicate china is put on a high shelf. Similarly the strain on both the child and others may be lessened by rearranging the immediate surroundings. At school, Paul, who would pull the hair of any child within reach, was placed at a desk well away from the rest of the class. This did not teach him not to pull hair but it did allow him to learn other things, and to be reinforced for it, without the learning being constantly interrupted by hair pulling. Later, as he was enjoying what he was doing, and the reinforcement, it became possible to move him gradually nearer to the other children.

This 'avoidance–prevention' tactic sounds obvious but it is worth remembering as another available strategy. Wherever possible it should not be seen as an end in itself, but, as in Paul's case, as providing an opportunity for the child to be taught, to learn, and to make progress that in time will help to make the avoidance strategy unnecessary.

I shall now turn to ways of tackling the behaviour itself.

Encouraging better behaviours
The full title for this method is 'differential reinforcement of other behaviours', or DRO for short. With it, the undesirable behaviour is tackled by encouraging another, positive behaviour to take its place. Often the behaviour encouraged is one that makes it impossible for the child to be carrying out the undesirable behaviour at the same time—the two are incompatible. This is often known as 'differential reinforcement of incompatible behaviours', or DRI. Carol had poor sight and had further damaged her eyes by poking them with her fingers. She was very fond of loud squeaky noises, so a piece of apparatus was constructed for her which, when a switch was pressed, produced these sounds. She was reinforced by the squeaky noises for pressing the switch, and she could only do this if she were not poking her eyes—or so it was thought. In fact, Carol proved remarkably resourceful in finding ways in which she could do both at once, and it was only when the apparatus was finally adapted

so that she had to press two sets of switches at the same time with her fingertips, that pressing for the sounds and eye-poking became truly incompatible. She loved the apparatus and would use it whenever she could, so after this there were long stretches of time when she was not damaging her eyes.

This is a rather specific example, and in many cases DRO is more straightforward. The child can be reinforced for simply *not* doing the behaviour. Seven-year-old Wilfred's problem was aggression: he would hit, kick or scratch the other children at school, and his brother and sister at home. When he did this at school he was taken out of class and sent to sit in the headmaster's room, and during this time he seemed quite subdued . His behaviour, however, did not improve. When his mother sought help she reported, "He had been taken out of class three times by 10.30 this morning"—not only was this approach not reducing the behaviour, it might even have been increasing it. Everyone got together to work out a better plan. There were a number of treats that Wilfred very much enjoyed—playing football with his father, going for walks in the woods, and going swimming. It was decided to divide his day up into four periods: before school, the morning up until lunchtime, after lunch until the end of school, and the rest of the afternoon and evening until bedtime. For each of these periods in which Wilfred had not hit, kicked or scratched anyone he got a sticker, and when he had four stickers—whether or not they were collected over a single day—he could choose to have one of his treats. Wilfred looked forward to the treats so much that his aggression got less and less; because he did not hit them, the other children became more friendly to him; and in time the programme could be discontinued.

MAKING SURE WE ARE NOT ENCOURAGING UNDESIRABLE BEHAVIOURS

Nobody encourages undesirable behaviours on purpose, but this can come about accidentally. As discussed earlier, a behaviour can be encouraged by reinforcing it. This is the aim for positive behaviours—learning skills or becoming more cooperative. Sometimes, however, it may become apparent that reinforcement is following a behaviour that is not wanted at all: this is usually because it had not been realized that what followed *was* a reinforcer. When Vincent called a visitor "Fat lady!" his mother sternly ticked him off. Vincent smiled broadly and repeated, "Fat lady! Fat lady!" His mother had intended the ticking-off to put a stop to his name-calling; his reaction suggested instead that it encouraged him to do it again. Often these inadvertent reinforcers are found to be connected to the attention the child's behaviour obtains. The attention may consist of displeasure or anger, but for some children this is a great deal better than no attention at all.

When it becomes clear that a response is reinforcing the behaviour, albeit unintentionally, one obvious solution is to stop the reinforcer from following the behaviour. This strategy is known as *extinction*: provided that cessation of reinforcement is maintained, the behaviour will eventually die out (extinguish). Ann's mother was concerned about another of her behaviours, swearing. Ann would swear at her mother both when they were out and when they were at home—"She'll sit on the washing machine and swear at me." When Ann did this her mother felt upset, explained that it was rude and told her not to do it. When this had no effect her mother would give her a scolding, but Ann went on swearing. It seemed likely that all the attention that she got for her behaviour was reinforcing and maintaining it. So it was decided that in the future, when Ann swore, her mother would take no notice. This was quite hard for her to do at first. She and the psychologist had several rehearsals in which first the psychologist asked Ann's mother to swear at her, whereupon the psychologist looked mildly into the middle distance, remarked on the weather and said that perhaps they might go out in the afternoon. "Oh, I *see*," said Ann's mother, "you don't react *at all*." Then Ann's mother took a turn, the psychologist doing the swearing while she feigned nonchalence, and later she was able to do the same with Ann. Ann's swearing reduced quickly: she took to saying 'Oh blow', and everybody was happy.

Extinction can be a valuable strategy, but it needs careful consideration. First, it can only be used where the reinforcer can be controlled. If a child clowns around in the classroom and is reinforced by the laughter of the other children, it may be difficult to stop the reinforcer following the behaviour, and some method other than extinction may have to be looked for. (For example, we might reinforce *all* the children for times when the child was not clowning.)

Second, it is very important to know that, when extinction is put into practice, there is likely to be an initial *increase* in the behaviour. What seems to happen is this: the child does the behaviour, expecting the reinforcement; reinforcement does not appear; s/he tries again, and again. If the reinforcement still fails to appear s/he may increase the level of the behaviour, doing it louder or longer, more quickly or more violently. If the reinforcement is initially withheld but then, as the behaviour intensifies, resolution crumbles and the reinforcement is given, the situation is made worse. The child learns that, although s/he might not get the reinforcer straight away, s/he has only to keep the behaviour up long enough or do it more strenuously and reinforcement will come. Apart from anything else, this makes it much harder eventually to eliminate it. Thus before an extinction programme is begun, one must ask, can it be seen it through, and can the behaviour be coped with it if it gets worse? If the answer to both these questions is not a definite yes, extinction had better not even be attempted.

Third, the effect extinction will have on the child's life needs to be considered. By definition, extinction involves the child being deprived of reinforcement (for the unwanted behaviour), so wherever possible a parallel programme in which s/he is given reinforcement for desirable behaviour is set up. Chrissie's parents wanted to help her to cut down her constant, inappropriate crying. They realized that when she cried they had been paying her a great deal of attention, so they determined they would no longer do that. At the same time they saw that hitherto, whenever she was *not* crying, they had left her alone—understandably, they had grabbed any of the all-too-infrequent gaps between her crying spells to do something else. Now, however, while they ignored any crying that did not have a good reason for it, they also made strenuous efforts to pay attention to her when she was *not* crying. Non-crying was reinforced (DRO) and crying was not (extinction), and together these two programmes resulted in a much more cheerful, confident little girl and a much happier family.

When the child does not just forfeit reinforcement for inappropriate behaviours but also gets it for positive behaviours, it becomes less likely that the undesirable behaviours will return or be replaced by others. By supplying the child with reinforcement for the desirable behaviours it becomes unnecessary for her/him to seek this by other means.

'TIME OUT' (TIME OUT FROM POSITIVE REINFORCEMENT)

If, when a child who is in an enjoyable (reinforcing) situation exhibits an undesirable or inappropriate behaviour, the reinforcement is removed for a short while, then the child experiences 'time out' from the reinforcement. Subsequently the reinforcement is reintroduced, and removed again only if the behaviour reoccurs. Through the repeated association of the behaviour with the loss of reinforcement the child comes to understand that the one brings about the other, and s/he is likely to show less and less of the unwanted behaviour.

Don, 12 years old and with severe physical and learning disabilities, was very fond of music. He could not dress himself, so his mother dressed him every morning, switching on the radio for him to listen to. Don had got into the way of being awkward to dress, going into giggles and deliberately stiffening his arms and legs when his mother tried to get them into the garments. So she decided to use time out from the reinforcer—the music. When Don made it difficult to put the garment on she switched the music off for 15 seconds. Don found he got more enjoyment from the music if he did not make the dressing difficult, and dressing became an easier and more pleasant time for both of them.

Time out can be used with almost any reinforcer that is continuously available to the child and, as with extinction, is under outside control. Mealtime problems can be treated by briefly removing the child's plate—if, that is, s/he is very fond of the food. Removing the plate would not be much use with a child who did not like food. Trevor was very, very fond of his food, so much so that he would eat it far too fast, piling in one mouthful after another and often abandoning his cutlery and eating with his fingers —even things like stew, mashed potatoes and jelly. So every time Trevor gobbled or used his fingers his plate was removed for 10 seconds. In a remarkably short time he learned to eat more elegantly, finishing one mouthful before taking another and using his cutlery instead of his fingers.

Time out can be used very effectively when the reinforcers are the social ones—smiles, hugs and kisses, attention or just being in company. Time out from this kind of reinforcer may consist in walking or turning away from the child, or simply turning away the head. Then, when the behaviour has stopped for a few moments the child is attended to once more. Time out has often been associated with putting the child in another room, but it does not have to involve that. It can come in many other forms, and the use of 'time-out rooms' has lost favour now because of the possibility of this leading to abuse. Furthermore, in many programmes purporting to use 'time-out rooms' it was clear that what was being used was not 'time out' at all. Remember the full title, 'time out from positive reinforcement': it can only be expected to work if what is removed when the behaviour occurs is really a reinforcer. So, for a time-out room to work, the child has to value what it is s/he is being removed from. This was in fact the case with Fergus. Fergus had frequent temper tantrums in which he kicked and bit his mother. After some discussion she decided that, when he did that, he would be put in his bedroom until he was quiet for 30 seconds. His bedroom was full of his toys, apart from his tape recorder which his mother removed when she put him in the room. Over the weeks Fergus's tantrums diminished. Although his bedroom was a pleasant place, what he lost when he was in there was his mother's company, and this was enough for him to stop the kicking and biting. However, if a child actually dislikes being with other people, then brief periods of isolation can prove very reinforcing.

STIMULUS CONTROL

Much of everyday life is influenced by signals coming from the surroundings. A pedestrian walks to the edge of a pavement, and if s/he sees a green light ahead s/he crosses the road. A person starts towards the front door but if s/he sees rain falling outside s/he goes back and fetches a mackintosh or umbrella. The green light signals that crossing the road should be safe; the rain, that it would not be a good idea to go out unprotected—if it were falling in torrents that might be a signal not to go out at all. The signals suggest what behaviours will be successful (reinforced) and what will not. In the same way it may be possible to establish signals that will tell the child when a behaviour is acceptable (will be reinforced) and when it is not (will not be reinforced). S/he is shown when, and under what conditions, the behaviour will be permitted. As with 'free-star fining' this means that the behaviour is sometimes allowed, and so is not a suitable method for dangerous behaviours. It can, however, be used for non-dangerous, tiresome behaviours, or for behaviours that we want to reduce but not necessarily get rid of altogether.

Robert's behaviour was a good example. He presented his teachers with a range of problems of such severity that they asked for help from a psychologist. At the meeting called to discuss the problems, of the 11 listed it was decided to focus on one, question-asking. Robert would ask questions obsessively, often picking on a teacher who was obviously busy, standing in front of the teacher, repeating the question over and over again, or, if the question were answered, going on to question that as well. Although some of his other problems were more alarming (threatening to jab people in the eyes, ripping up clothing and curtains) the teachers felt that many of these followed on from the questioning and his agitation that resulted from that. They decided to try stimulus control. Robert was given a coloured sticker to wear on his jumper, and told that so long as he was wearing the sticker his questions would be answered. When the sticker was removed the questions would not be answered. The sticker on his jumper was a signal, 'Questions will be answered'. The programme was at first set up to run only between 9 and 10 a.m., and the sticker was removed for four 15 second periods. On the first day, when the sticker was removed, Robert bombarded the staff with questions, but they told him, "No, you haven't got your sticker, wait till you get it back." After this first day his attempts at questioning reduced rapidly over the eight weeks of the programme until there were none in the last four weeks. At the same time the teachers noticed that even when he was wearing the sticker he would, if staff were busy, wait until they were less busy to ask a question. Overall the number of questions he asked became fewer, with a decrease, too, in the other 'follow-on' problems. Although it was originally planned to extend the programme to more of the day, because of the change in Robert's behaviour generally this was not necessary.

Conclusions

Behavioural methods are not the answer to all the needs of children with learning disabilities. Many other aspects of their lives will have to be addressed—friendships and social relationships; their development into adulthood; their place in and rights as members of society—and many other methods and approaches will be necessary. Nevertheless, behavioural methods, applied thoughtfully and sensitively, and always tailored to the needs of the individual child, can often help. For some problems, as I have outlined in this chapter, they may be the main method used; for others they may be found valuable in conjunction with and in support of any other appropriate method. They are there to be used, or not, as the situation requires.

REFERENCES

Premack, D. (1959) 'Toward empirical behavior laws. 1. Positive reinforcement.' *Psychological Review*, **66**, 219–233.

Salend, S.J., Kovalich, B. (1965) 'A group response–cost system mediated by free tokens: an alternative to token reinforcement.' *American Journal of Mental Deficiency*, **86**, 748-751.

FURTHER READING

Carr, J. (1995) *Helping Your Handicapped Child: a Step-by-Step Guide to Everyday Problems. 2nd Edn.* Harmondsworth: Penguin.

Durand, V.M., Carr, E.G. (1991) 'Functional communication training to reduce challenging behavior: maintenance and application in new settings.' *Journal of Applied Behavior Analysis*, **24**, 251–264.

Donnellan, A.M., LaVigna, G.W., Negri-Schoultz, N., Fassbender, L.L. (1988) *Progress Without Punishment.* New York and London: Teacher's College Press.

Emerson, E. (1993) 'Challenging behaviours and severe learning disabilities: recent developments in behavioural analysis and intervention.' *Behavioural and Cognitive Psychotherapy*, **21**, 171–198.

Kazdin, A.E. (1975) *Behavior Modification in Applied Settings.* Homewood, IL: Dorsey Press.

Murphy, G., Wilson, B. (1985) *Self-injurious behaviour: a Collection of Published Papers on Prevalence, Causes and Treatment in People Who are Mentally Handicapped or Autistic.* Kidderminster: BIMH Publications.

Yule, W., Carr, J. (1987) *Behaviour Modification for People with Mental Handicaps, 2nd Edn.* London: Croom Helm.

Zarkowska, E., Clements, J. (1988) *Problem Behaviour in People with Severe Learning Difficulties: a Practical Guide to a Constructional Approach.* London: Croom Helm.

5
COMMUNICATION AND LANGUAGE DISORDERS

Ilene S. Schwartz, Ann N. Garfinkle, Gail Joseph and Bonnie J. McBride

A schoolgirl using a secret code to tell her best friend about what happened in science class . . .
An athletics coach calling plays by holding up three fingers . . .
A man placing an order at a restaurant for lunch . . .
A businesswoman sending an associate electronic mail about the latest merger . . .
A toddler stretching out his arms when his father walks into the room . . .

The above events are everyday examples of how, without even thinking about it, we use a variety of forms of communication to express a variety of different types of information, for a variety of different reasons, with a variety of partners, and to accomplish a variety of objectives. In fact, almost all of our daily behavior is communicative. Functional communication consists of those behaviors and skills that enable us to obtain our needs and wants, to influence or change the behaviors of others, and to relate to one another in an enjoyable way.

Traditionally, communication has been divided into five areas of study: phonology, morphology, semantics, syntax, and pragmatics. These categories are useful because they help to organize communication in such a way that it can be understood as a generalized system and may be helpful in determining specific interventions for individual skill deficits. However, they may actually serve as a barrier to facilitating a functional communication system for children with global delays. An alternative conceptualization is to think of communication in terms of form, content, and use.

The form of communication refers to the manner by which the message is delivered: form is *how* we communicate. The most commonly used form is speech because it is generally efficient and effective. There is, however, a range of other acceptable and effective forms, including American Sign Language (ASL). Codes, conventional gestures and written words are also common, as the brief examples above illustrate. In addition, a number of alternative or augmentative forms of communication are often used with children with disabilities, including the Picture Exchange Communication System (PECS) (Bondy and Frost 1994), symbol systems and computerized communication systems. In the wake of important research in the field of developmental disabilities (*e.g.* Carr and Durand 1985), researchers and practitioners are beginning to recognize challenging behavior (*e.g.* aggression, self-injury, property destruction) as a form of communication. Through a series of elegant experiments, Carr and Durand demonstrated that by strengthening more appropriate forms of communication, the inappropriate forms (*i.e.* the challenging behaviors) decrease.

Understanding inappropriate behavior as a form of communication is an important first step in decreasing such behavior and helping to develop a functional communication system (Koegel *et al.* 1996). Nevertheless, the particular form of the communication (as long as it is appropriate) is not nearly as important as the content or function of the communication (Skinner 1957).

Content is *what* is being communicated. In the examples above, the science lesson, the team's play, the food order, the business news and wanting to be picked up are what is being communicated. In each of these, the people communicating have desires, needs and information that they want to share. In order for the content to be understood, however, the recipient must be able to recognize the form of the message and understand enough about the content (*i.e.* have some experience or knowledge of the content) in order to interpret the meaning of the communication. In order to be a successful communicator, there must be things in your environment about which you want and need to communicate. For many children with disabilities, people in their environment may preempt this by anticipating their wants and needs, or the environment itself may be so sterile that they literally have nothing to talk about. Experience in an interesting and stimulating environment provides content for communication and thus facilitates functional communication.

Use of communication is the ability to select an appropriate form to frame its content so that the recipient understands the message. In the above examples, we do not know if the schoolgirl, the athletics coach, the man, the businesswoman or the toddler have been successful in their attempts to communicate. If the schoolgirl's friend understands the science lesson, if the player understands what to do, if the man gets his lunch, if the business associate understands the news, and if the toddler gets picked up, then their use of communication was successful. Success depends on the interaction between the communicative partners. Thus, children with disabilities need to learn to be successful as both speaker and listener, and to communicate with a wide variety of partners.

In fact, effective communication can only take place when the communicator is competent in the employment of form, content and use (Wetherby and Prizant 1990), and these concepts may therefore be more useful than the traditional systems of categorization when planning interventions. Nevertheless, these two forms of conceptualization are not mutually exclusive. For example, if we discover that a child's communicative attempts are largely unsuccessful due to extremely poor articulation, we can view this as a problem in form, and specifically as a phonological problem. By using these frameworks interactively, we can begin articulation therapy and work with the child to use other forms (*e.g.* pointing, gestures, or pictures) to augment her/his communication. This view of communication emphasizes the interactional as well as the structural components of communication.

It is important to note, however, that there is no magic standard for the level of competence in form, content and use that one must master in order to be viewed as a competent communicator. Because communication is a process of sharing information, the level of competence that one must exhibit to communicate effectively is determined, in part, by the persistence and adaptability of the speaker, the sophistication of the communicative partner, the familiarity of the situation and content, the complexity of the message, and a number of other complex interactional variables.

The social context of communication

To understand the idea that communication is a dynamic process between communicator and partner, it is also crucial to understand the role of the wider social context. Social context includes the people who are communicating, the environment in which they are communicating, the community in which one typically communicates, and the role(s) that one plays within these settings.

It may be helpful to understand that every social context is related to a social community or culture that has its own norms and traditions. The meaning is agreed on, implicitly or explicitly, by the community, and therefore the competence of any communicative inter-action or of an individual communicator must be viewed through these cultural lenses (Moerk 1992).

For children the most important social context is the family because of the role it plays in development. It is within the social context of the family that children have some of their most salient experiences with communication—both as communicators and as communicative partners. In an extensive study of children's learning, Hart and Risley (1995) demonstrated that the child's experience in the home in the first three years of life had a tremendous effect on development. Specifically, children who were involved in many warm and friendly communication acts had better long-term developmental outcomes than children who had fewer, more negative communication experiences. Outcome was strongly related to the types of language environment to which the children were exposed, and these in turn were strongly related to the socioeconomic status of the families. These differences were long-lasting and affected many aspects of the child's life, in particular their expressive vocabularies and performance in school (Walker *et al.* 1994).

Children with difficulties, delays or disorders in communication are at a disadvantage in many other areas of development as well. For example, they may have short attention spans (Baker and Cantwell 1982), difficulty with reading (Silva *et al.* 1987), behavioral problems, or difficulty with social adjustment (Aram and Hall 1989). This broad-reaching effect is the reason that communication is often described as a 'pivotal behavior' (Koegel and Frea 1993). Because of this it is very important that children learn to communicate as effectively as possible. When delays or disorders in communication skills occur, intervention is required (Nye *et al.* 1987, Olswang and Bain 1991, Guralnick 1997, McLean and Cripe 1997).

There are many excellent resources for planning interventions for children with disabilities (*e.g.* Bailey and Wolery 1992, Bricker and Cripe 1992, Freeman and Dake 1997). While the specifics of many programs vary, we would like to suggest some general criteria to follow when planning interventions (Table 5.1), and some guidelines that can be used to help families evaluate their effectiveness (Table 5.2). As described above, communication is a complex and culturally bound behavior. This complexity often requires a multifaceted approach to intervention (Warren and Yoder 1994). It also makes designing, implementing and evaluating interventions extremely challenging. This daunting task is made easier, however, with a basic understanding of communication, the ability to work collaboratively with family members and other caregivers, and knowledge of behavioral instructional strategies.

TABLE 5.1
Guidelines for intervention

- Family members should be invited to participate as members of the intervention team
- All decisions should be made in collaboration with the family
- Interventions must be culturally responsive and respectful
- The needs and priorities of the family should drive the intervention
- The types of intervention strategies selected and the location of the intervention should be based upon the needs of the child
- The goals, contexts and strategies of intervention should be effective, efficient, functional and normalized (Bailey and McWilliam 1990)
- The intervention should result in functional, generalized behavior change

TABLE 5.2
Guiding questions for families

- Are the goals and objectives stated clearly and are they important to you?
- Are the procedures of the intervention clearly stated and are they acceptable to you?
- Are the procedures based on strategies that have been documented in the research literature?
- Do the data collected on your child convince you that this strategy is working?
- How does this procedure affect your family and is this acceptable to you?

What we know about facilitating communication skills

The field of behavioral communication intervention has changed dramatically in the last 30 years. Whereas in the first issue of the *Journal of Applied Behavior Analysis*, published in 1968, most of the research questions were concerned with attempting to understand if behaviors could be changed and what strategies were effective to facilitate these changes, most of the current behavioral literature is interested in how these changes can be generalized to everyday environments and how researchers can work with teachers, parents and child care providers to implement these strategies. These changes are reflected in an article by Goldstein and Hockenberger (1991) in which they reviewed language intervention articles published between 1978 and 1988. Five themes emerged from this literature: the development of augmentative/alternative communication systems; teaching children to take advantage of observational learning opportunities; teaching a variety of communicative functions; teaching language as a means of self and environmental control; and study of facilitating generalization. The authors emphasized that communication is a pivotal skill, and intervention is best embedded in a relevant social context utilizing key personnel relevant to that context (*e.g.* peers and family members). They also suggest that effective interventions will systematically plan for generalization.

The emphasis on teaching communication skills in relevant social contexts has resulted in a focus on 'naturalistic' language strategies. Warren *et al.* (1980) identified three components common to all these types of interventions: creating a need for communication in the environment, making communication functional, and reinforcing all language use. Hepting and Goldstein (1996) identified 11 specific intervention strategies involved in naturalistic interventions: prompting imitation; 'mand' (see below); requesting clarification or elaboration; waiting for a response; environmental arrangement; modeling; repeating and recasting; descriptive talking; delivering desired consequences; praise; and minimal encouragement. There are few data, however, that indicate which of these strategies is most effective or how to match specific strategies to specific children or disorders (Guralnick 1997). There are also questions about the extent to which these strategies are actually used in early childhood settings. In two large classroom-based studies, Schwartz et al. (1996) examined the frequency with which identified best practices were used, and the relationship between the use of these recommended practices and child engagement and language growth. They found that there was huge variation in the type of language intervention that occurred across classrooms, but that in classrooms in which teachers implemented recommended strategies children demonstrated higher rates of active engagement and made greater gains on language measures.

In one of the few studies that have attempted to compare the relative effectiveness of language intervention strategies, Nye et al. (1987) used a meta-analysis technique to review 48 research articles, concentrating on those that employed imitation, elicitation, modeling, focused stimulation, compression and psychosocial techniques. The modeling approach was reported as the most effective. However, these techniques were most likely to improve the *syntax* of a target child; pragmatics were not generally affected. The authors also reported that standardized methods of measurement did not show the amount of improvement that was revealed by the analysis of language samples.

A number of studies have examined the role of the environment and social context in teaching communication skills (Hemmeter and Kaiser 1990), and it is clear that intervention can be made more effective by making appropriate changes to the environment. Koegel (1995) emphasizes that when providing language treatment to children a meaningful context is essential, and suggests that the more atypical a situation is, the less the skills taught will generalize to other contexts. She reminds therapists that children use language most fully when there is something important that they want to communicate about; thus, the therapist should not impose the content of conversation on the child. These studies and others (for excellent reviews, see Klinger and Dawson 1992, Sainato and Carta 1992) demonstrate the importance of a supportive social–communicative context and an interesting environment in planning effective communication interventions.

Although much of the behavioral communication research in the last decade has consisted of a hybrid of 'naturalistic' techniques, most of the approaches that have been developed stem from three primary strategies: mand model, time delay, and incidental teaching. Each of these is described in greater detail below, but briefly: mand model is an adult-initiated strategy that teaches students to respond to questions and to instructions for verbalizations (Rogers-Warren and Warren 1980), the aim being to increase general responsiveness and to teach new vocabulary items; the time-delay procedure (Halle et al. 1979) teaches students to initiate language by responding to nonspeech, environmental prompts and is best used to increase spontaneity and to decrease students' reliance on verbal prompts; and incidental teaching (Hart and Risley 1968, 1974, 1975, 1980) is a child-initiated technique with adults using a child's initiation as an opportunity to request an expansion or elaboration, and is most appropriate when teaching students to use more complex and longer utterances. These strategies have been expanded and modified to meet the needs of diverse learners—for excellent reviews, see Hepting and Goldstein (1996) and Kaiser *et al.* (1992).

This brief review suggests that there are many effective language-intervention strategies available. The challenge continues to be in how we match the appropriate strategy to the needs of the child and family. Assessment, therefore, is a crucial preliminary stage in the development of any intervention program.

Assessment of language and communication skills
DIMENSIONS OF ASSESSMENT

Traditionally, language and communication assessment has focused on the child's level of communication and the degree of comprehension of speech (Prizant and Schuler 1987). However, it is now recognized that this is only one dimension and that a comprehensive communication assessment needs to address a child's skills in communicative use as well as identifying the behavioral aspects of learning environments and communication partners that support or limit successful communicative exchange.

Assessing child skills
Specific dimensions of a child's communicative content, form and use should be assessed to provide a profile of communicative strengths and identify appropriate targets for intervention. Specific content areas that should be assessed are: (1) expressive language and communication; (2) receptive language and communication; (3) speech production or primary communication mode (*e.g.* sign, symbol); (4) language-related cognitive skills; and (5) social-affective behavior.

Assessing learning environments
As noted above, physical and social aspects of the environment play an important role in the development of communicative competence (Rogers-Warren *et al.* 1983, Hart and Risley 1995). Thus the availability of materials in the environment as well as the child's need to use language skills should also be considered as part of a comprehensive assessment. Aspects of the physical environment include the selection and arrangement of materials, the arrangement of the setting to encourage the child's engagement, and scheduling of activities to support the child's participation and appropriate behavior. Essential aspects of the social environment include the presence of communicative partners and the verbal and nonverbal social interactions that occur among them.

Assessing the skills of the communicative partner
Communicative partners (*e.g.* parents, other family members and caregivers, educators, therapists, peers, community members) demonstrate a wide range of behaviors that may support or in some cases hinder a child's communicative development (Field 1987). A communicative partner's skill in supporting communicative transactions may be assessed during observations of daily routines and play activities. Dimensions of partner style include level of acceptance of a child's communicative attempts (Duchan 1989), use of directive

versus facilitative modes of interaction (Duchan 1989, Marfo 1990), and use of specific strategies such as responding contingently to child behavior, provision of appropriate communicative models, maintaining the topics of child initiations, and expanding or elaborating on communicative attempts (Peck 1989).

Assessing partner style is predicated on the aim of helping partners develop an awareness of the strategies they are using. This is especially important for children with augmentative systems, non-standard communicative forms, or poor articulation. While there is no single ideal communicative style for *all* children and partners, factors such as a child's developmental level, previous communicative experiences, and social motivation all need to be taken into account. A partner's degree of comfort using a certain style and the familial and cultural influences on interactions with children must also be considered.

ASSESSMENT GUIDELINES

In the section above we have outlined the type of information that should be included in a comprehensive communication assessment. Now we present three guidelines that can be used by practitioners to frame their assessment practices.

• *Guideline #1: Assessment is an ongoing process. A variety of assessment types and procedures should be utilized for collecting information. These should be selected according to the child's developmental level and the purpose of the assessment, as well as what the family wants, needs and finds useful.*

Different forms of assessment provide different information and it is crucial that the assessment types and procedures employed match specific needs for information as well as the family's priorities. For example, most norm-referenced tests yield results that do not help in planning appropriate and meaningful intervention. On the other hand, they do provide information about the child's development compared to a normative sample and this is important for identifying children who need specialized instruction. The three most widely used methods of assessment are direct test, behavioral observation, and parent/caregiver interview or report.

Direct testing is utilized when the professional wants to know how a child responds to a standardized stimulus, a request or a specific set of materials (Bailey 1989), and involves standardized administration procedures, materials and interpretation of the results. There are three different types of direct tests: norm-referenced, criterion-referenced, and curriculum-referenced or curriculum-based assessment.

The major purpose of the norm-referenced test is to help therapists see how a child compares with other students of the same age or class placement. Norm-referenced tests yield at least four types of scores that provide a basis for comparing a child's performance with that of a normative population: developmental age scores, developmental quotients, standard scores and percentile ranks. Information derived from norm-referenced tests is usually required to determine a child's eligibility for services.

Criterion-referenced tests are composed of items selected because of their importance to daily living or school performance. Criterion-referenced tests indicate ability with respect to specific skills rather than provide information about where a child's performance is relative to her/his peers.

Curriculum-referenced testing or curriculum-based assessment tells us what skills the child has acquired and where the child is in comparison to a curriculum. These assessments offer behavioral and concrete information that aids in developing appropriate intervention programs.

Behavioral observation can yield an eclectic collection of valid, reliable information, and does not constrain the child's behavior or limit their competence. A behavioral observation is a recording of a child's behavior across a variety of settings, within a variety of contexts and with multiple communicative partners. This approach provides additional information about how (*e.g.* independent, with verbal prompts) a child performs certain behaviors, and can be extremely helpful when planning interventions.

Interviewing parents and primary caregivers is useful when professionals are collecting information about the family's perceptions of their child's skills and their priorities for intervention. Interviews can be either structured or open-ended, allowing the interviewer to pursue areas of concern as they arise.

Each of these procedures provides qualitatively different information about a child's communicative abilities. While they can be used together to construct an holistic picture of a child's communication system, none alone provides a complete picture. The utilization of multiple methods of assessment allows for triangulation of findings and can contribute to the overall reliability and validity of the process. For a detailed listing and discussion of communication assessment instruments, see Rosetti (1990) and Crais and Roberts (1996).

• *Guideline #2: Great importance should be placed on parents and primary caregivers as expert informants about their child's communication skills.*

The appropriateness of communication skills must be evaluated within an appropriate cultural context. Without information from the families it is extremely difficult to collect adequate assessment information or interpret those results appropriately. Within the area of communication skills, parents, caregivers and others familiar with the child can often provide unique insights into the form, content and use of the child's communication system as well as the best strategies to engage the child in interaction. Parents and caregivers see children in a far wider array of situations and over more extended periods of time than is possible for any professional. Moreover, involving parents in the assessment of their child conveys a message that their information is valued and respected. Parents and caregivers can participate in assessment via interviews as well as by completing standardized measurements, rating scales and checklists or by conducting behavioral observations. Research has documented the high reliability of parent reporting (Bricker and Squires 1989, Dale *et al.* 1989, Dale 1991). Parents may also be a valuable resource for interpreting the results of an assessment in a culturally meaningful way.

• *Guideline #3: Assessment should always provide direct implications and directions for intervention, and lead directly to ongoing evaluation.*

A systems approach to intervention actively links assessment to intervention and evaluation activities. In particular, a linked system utilizes the information acquired during the assessment to develop intervention goals (Bricker 1993, 1996). The intervention goals, in turn, guide the selection of intervention content and strategies. Evaluation of a child's progress is focused on attainment of goals and is congruent with the assessment procedures.

In other words, the assessment process should produce the necessary information to select appropriate and meaningful intervention targets (Schwartz and Olswang 1996). Again, the formal inclusion of input from parents and caregivers will facilitate the development of appropriate, realistic and meaningful intervention goals.

Strategies for intervention
Once a thorough communication assessment has been conducted, the question of how and when to intervene must be addressed. The strategies presented below are adapted from the *Project ECLIPSE Curriculum: Classroom Strategies for Promoting the Communicative Independence of Young Children with Disabilities* (Schwartz et al. 1993)*. The goal of this curriculum is to enable teachers, child-care providers and families to improve the communication skills of children with disabilities (Schwartz *et al.* 1996) and to promote the communicative independence of each child. 'Communicative independence' is the child's ability to conduct meaningful and functional exchanges with other people, respond to others, and maintain communicative interactions.

A critical component of teaching the functional use of language (in whatever form) is to identify naturally occurring opportunities throughout the day and to create others to ensure that a child has many opportunities within different environments and with different communicative partners to practice her/his communication skills.

The naturalistic teaching strategies described below share several common components: (1) teaching opportunities capitalize on children's interests; (2) multiple naturally occurring opportunities are used to teach language forms; (3) child communication is explicitly taught; (4) reinforcement relies on the natural consequences of the child's communication; (5) teaching episodes are embedded into the natural flow and routine of interactions.

The remainder of this section will focus on three components of a comprehensive intervention approach for promoting functional communication skills. The first two components (the social communicative context and the instructional environment) include specific techniques that can be used to provide a learning environment that is responsive and supportive of a child's communication attempts, and at the same time will promote independence within a variety of environments. The final component describes direct assist strategies for teaching specific language and communication forms, content and uses. However, these direct instructional strategies are meant to be phased out as a child's communication becomes more independent and more affected by the social context and naturally occurring opportunities in the environment.

THE SOCIAL COMMUNICATIVE CONTEXT
The social communicative context is the environment in which a child interacts with others, and is the foundation for building communicative independence. These environments must be especially sensitive to a child's attempts to communicate, and must encourage and reinforce all communicative attempts, even if they are difficult to interpret. In this context, the adult and the child become partners who share responsibility for selecting and maintaining

*For a complete copy of the curriculum, please contact the first author.

conversational topics and structures. Principles to facilitate a supportive social communicative context are described below.

• *Read child behavior as intent to interact.* Even before a child uses conventional means to communicate s/he will successfully use a variety of other behaviors (*e.g.* pointing, crying, motor movements). Children with developmental delays may use signals that are not easily interpretable as intentional communication or they may have difficulty responding to signals from others. The ability of an adult to interpret the child's communicative acts will help that child understand the relationship between her/his communication and the social environment. There are three components of this strategy that are important to consider.

First, *identify* consistent signals of communicative intent. As the child's communicative partner it is important to observe behavior that indicates child interest in materials, activities or people. Second, *react consistently* to communication signals. Using familiar, repeated and contextually linked responses to a child's communicative acts will increase the likelihood that the child will understand the link between her/his behavior and the impact it has on the social environment. Third, *comment* about the child's behavior using a conventional form (*e.g.* verbalizations, pictorial representation, sign and/or gestures). This provides the child with examples of conventional signals interpretable by a wide array of people. Providing new forms to replace the child's early unconventional forms of communication helps to increase her/his independence and ability to communicate with a wider variety of partners.

• *Establish joint attention.* The ability to establish and maintain attention between communicative partners is an important component of the social nature of communication. Paying attention to whatever activity the child shows interest in ensures that you and the child are focused on the same person, object or event. This strategy establishes a shared focus; by following the child's lead, you ensure that the child is engaged and interested in the topic, which in turn ensures participation and encourages continuing interaction. Although most children learn this without specific instruction, some children with communication disorders, especially children with autism, may need systematic instruction to develop this behavior (Tager-Flusberg 1989).

The first component of this strategy is identifying objects, activities and interactions that engage the child. Observe the child with a variety of materials or activities and systematically record her/his preferences or ask caregivers to identify highly preferred materials or activities. Then, express interest in the child's focus. Do this by commenting, gesturing or vocalizing interest and by orienting physically to the object of the child's interest with eye contact and physical proximity.

• *Provide opportunity for child input.* Exchange of information between conversational partners depends on turn-taking. Although this sounds simple, adults often preempt children's opportunities to talk (Schwartz *et al.* 1989). The key component of this strategy is being quiet and waiting (it is recommended at least five seconds) for the child to respond. This may seem counterintuitive to an adult who is accustomed to initiating and maintaining conversations, but it is an important step in teaching the social rules of communication. The amount of 'wait time' will vary depending on situational demands. If the child is in a familiar and routine situation in which s/he has adequate skills to initiate a comment or request then a longer pause for her/him to take the lead would be appropriate. In contrast, in a novel setting with unfamiliar materials or activities, the child might not be expected to initiate; instead the adult would provide time for the child to respond to modeled comments appropriate to the situation.

• *Respond actively and quickly to child's communicative attempts.* Responding to a child's communication in a timely and contingent manner will influence both the quantity and quality of communicative attempts. A response that is timely is a response that immediately follows the communicative message of the child. A contingent adult response is related to the topic initiated by the child, and acknowledges the child's questions, comments and requests.

• *Structuring opportunities for peer interaction.* An important component of promoting a child's communicative independence is providing opportunities for interaction with peers. These opportunities can occur in school, community and home settings. However, proximity to peers alone will not necessarily lead to meaningful or sustained contacts and it may be necessary to create opportunities for interaction and actively to support these.

Facilitating and supporting peer interactions requires careful planning. This could include the incorporation of activities that require the involvement of more than one child; providing enough materials for several children to work at the same time; and including materials that promote cooperative play such as sociodramatic play props and/or games.

Creating a facilitative instructional environment

An environment that lacks reinforcers and items of interests, or one that meets children's needs without requiring communicative attempts, is not a functional environment for learning or teaching language (Ostrosky and Kaiser 1991). Children must have reasons to communicate, such as the need to obtain assistance or request desired objects as well as to reject or protest in socially acceptable ways (Prizant and Schuler 1987, Peck 1989). Contexts in which children have shared control of the environment through decision making and choices have been associated with higher degrees of communicative initiation and spontaneity in older children with disabilities (Peck 1985, Houghton *et al.* 1987) and are now considered important in supporting communicative growth for young children (Theodore *et al.* 1990).

The manner in which materials or activities are made available to a child can influence the degree to which an environment facilitates or requires a child to communicate. For example, adults can negate the need for communication by making everything in the environment readily available to the child or they can reduce the need for communication by not providing clear contingencies for language use, or by anticipating a child's need before s/he expresses one. Similarly, if the physical environment is devoid of interesting materials, the motivation to make comments or initiate interest will be diminished.

The most successful way an adult can arrange the environment to support the use of language and communication skills is by embedding language instruction into ongoing daily activities and routines and allowing children the opportunity to communicate. Specific strategies might include the following.

• *Store preferred items so they are visible but out of reach.* It is important to ensure that the materials are in fact highly preferred by the child, and that they are stored so that they are visible but just out of reach. The objective is to ensure that access to the toy, material or activity is contingent upon communication. However, it is also necessary to strike a balance between items a child needs to request and those s/he can access independently. The goal is to create meaningful opportunities for communication, not a frustrating environment.

- *'Forget' important materials.* Adults can increase communication by intentionally 'forgetting' materials needed to complete a project or by missing out an important component of a daily routine. In order for this strategy to be successful the child must be familiar enough with an activity or routine to recognize that a central component has been omitted.

- *Require the child to seek assistance.* Create situations in which a child needs to communicate a need for assistance in order to complete a task. For example, this might be accomplished by placing the items needed for a game or activity in a container that is too difficult for the child to open independently. It is important not to choose situations where the goal is independence.

- *Use joint action routines.* Joint action routines (JARs) are effective techniques for teaching language in a context that is natural and meaningful to the child. JARs can fall into the category of environmental strategies because a JAR can set the stage for using other language strategies. To establish these, an adult must have a goal or theme in mind. Identify and follow a predictable sequence of events (which can involve turn-taking), identify roles, establish joint attention on a repetitive task, and then plan for slight variations in the routine. The establishment of the routine alone does not necessarily enhance communication skills— it is the act of embedding communication in the routine that makes this an effective strategy.

DIRECT ASSIST STRATEGIES

The goal of direct teaching techniques is to teach new and complex forms of communication and, more importantly, to teach effective and appropriate communication functions. These strategies are designed to be easily used and incorporated into ongoing interactions. They provide a range of intervention options, and each varies in the amount of direct adult intervention required. The selection of a strategy depends on the amount of adult assistance necessary to support a specific interaction at a particular moment. The degree of support needed will vary across and within children, and may alter according to the child's developmental needs, the specific targeted language objective, the familiarity of the task, the familiarity of the communicative partner, and the child's motivation at that moment.

While the five strategies described below share common goals and many common components they differ in the amount and intensity of adult intervention required to support the desired communicative behavior (Fig. 5.1). Another common element of all of these strategies is that they rely on identifying and capitalizing on opportunities for meaningful communication. These opportunities may occur naturally or may be deliberately created, as previously discussed. The important element is to identify these opportunities and link them to a language-teaching interaction. While it is impossible to take advantage of all possible naturally occurring opportunities for language interaction, it is important to be deliberate about selecting opportunities that provide highly salient examples of the language goals and are most motivating to the child.

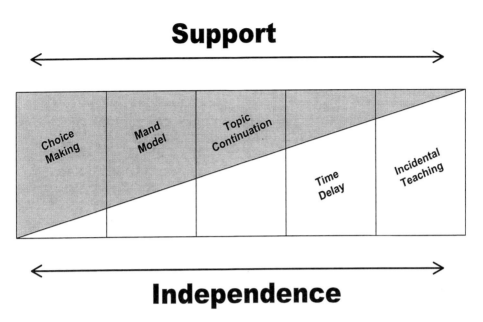

Fig. 5.1. Continuum of adult support and child independence across the five direct assist strategies.

• *Choice making.* This requires the highest degree of adult support. The adult initiates the interaction with the child by selecting the objects offered as choices. The goal of this strategy is to give the child the power to influence her/his environment through simple communicative behaviors—making a choice or voicing preference. This strategy is effective and practical with children who have a wide range of developmental needs and allows the child to gain control by acting on her/his environment (making a choice) in a meaningful way. Its logic is straightforward—a child is given the opportunity to select between two alternatives that are reasonable, available to the child, and of equal value. Identifying the most natural time within an activity that lends itself to offering a choice is the most efficient way in which to imbed this strategy, *e.g.* a choice between two preferred toys, or games, or food items at mealtimes.

Choice-making can be used effectively to meet diverse language goals. For example, it can be useful in teaching children to initiate conversations: present two choices, both appealing and interesting, and the material the child chooses can prompt the topic of conversation. This strategy is also useful with children who are working on single word utterances: offer the child a choice of two objects and use the object the child chooses as an opportunity to practice using that word by labelling the item chosen. Whatever the particular goal or outcome it is important always to reinforce the child's decision-making by giving her/him the requested object or activity, and supporting the implementation of this choice (*e.g.* if the child chooses a puzzle, provide as much support for her/him to play with the puzzle appropriately). Examples of interaction steps are shown in Table 5.3.

TABLE 5.3
Direct assist strategies

Step	Example
Choice making	During free choice in a preschool classroom, Bobby approaches the art area and inspects the different art materials. He sits down, takes a piece of paper and begins to draw with marker pens. He stops and looks at the other materials. He seems to be looking at the glue and the glitter. The teacher uses his interest in the glue to have him request that material.
1. Establish joint attention with the child by focusing the child's attention on what interests her/him at that moment.	
2. Present two options to the child and ask her/him to make a choice (*e.g.* "Do you want scissors or glue?").	
3. Provide an appropriate level of prompt if necessary to ensure a correct response.	
4. Confirm the child's response or give appropriate corrective feedback.	
5. Provide access to the requested material, information or activity contingent on an appropriate response.	
6. Keep the interaction brief.	
Mand model	Abby is standing in the hallway of her home waiting to go outside to play. She is holding her coat, but is having difficulty trying to put it on. Her mother takes advantage of this opportunity to have Abby ask for assistance. After Abby asks for help, she gets her coat on and goes outside.
1. Establish joint attention with the child by focusing the child's attention on what interests her/him at that moment.	
2. Give the child a verbal request (*e.g.* "Tell me what you want.")	
3. Give the child an opportunity to respond.	
4. Provide an appropriate level of prompt if necessary to ensure a correct response.	
5. Confirm the child's response or give appropriate corrective feedback.	
6. Provide access to the requested material, information or activity contingent on an appropriate response.	
7. Keep the interaction brief.	
Topic continuation	Anne is playing in the classroom with blocks and trains. She builds different structures and describes them for her teacher. Her teacher follows her lead and provides enough structure for Anne to be able to engage in another conversational turn.
1. Follow the child's conversational lead (*e.g.* child says, "I made a train station.")	
2. Respond to the child's turn using comments, questions or a script (adult responds, "How many trains will fit in the station?")	
3. Give the child an opportunity to respond.	
4. Confirm the child's response or give appropriate corrective feedback.	
5. Keep the interaction going.	
Time delay	At home, James sees his favorite cookies in a clear container on the counter. His mother blocks his access to the cookies and looks at him expectantly. James says, "Want cookie", and his mother gives him one.
1. Identify an appropriate opportunity.	
2. Block access to the desired material, object or activity.	
3. Do not vocalize, verbalize or sign to the child, while maintaining joint attention with the child.	
4. Maintain these conditions for at least 5 seconds or until the child responds.	
5. Provide an appropriate level of prompt if necessary to ensure a correct response.	
6. Confirm the child's response or give approopriate corrective feedback.	
7. Provide access to the requested material, information or activity contingent on an appropriate response.	
8. Keep the interaction brief.	
Incidental teaching	Ben is painting at the easel. He has yellow, green and red paint. He uses all the yellow paint and says to the teacher, "More paint." The teacher responds, "What kind of paint?" Ben responds, "Yellow." The teacher fills his container with yellow paint and he continues to paint.
1. Identify a child initiation as a teachable moment.	
2. Request an elaboration or expansion of the child's communicative behavior.	
3. Give the child an opportunity to respond.	
4. Provide an appropriate level of prompt if necessary to ensure a correct response.	
5. Respond in a positive manner to the child's response and provide access to the requested material, information or activity contingent on an appropriate response.	
6. Keep the interaction brief.	

• *Mand model.* This is an adult-initiated procedure that teaches the child to respond to questions and instructions for verbalizations (Rogers-Warren and Warren 1980). The adult targets a teaching opportunity by identifying a situation in which the child needs to make a request in order to obtain a desired object or activity. The adult begins the interaction by offering assistance in acquiring the desired item, contingent upon the use of a conventional form of communication (verbalization, sign, picture). If the child correctly requests the item or imitates the model (*i.e.* verbal model, sign or picture), the adult responds by giving the child access to the desired item. If the child does not respond correctly, a corrective model or physical support (signing or use of a picture) is given and a close approximation to the desired form of communication may be honored in order to avoid frustration for the child. This approach closely follows the components of a naturalistic teaching strategy in that it relies on the child's interest(s) to start the teaching episode, and reinforcement of the correct response is tied directly to the communication act (*i.e.* the child gets what s/he asked for) instead of to an arbitrary reinforcer.

• *Topic continuation.* This has two general goals—to increase a child's participation in conversational interactions, and to encourage use of multi-word replies. The strategy is designed to promote a child's investment in a conversation and keep her/him involved in the interaction. Topic continuation strategies are most appropriate for children who initiate conversations but have limited skills in maintaining them. When a child initiates a conversational interaction the teacher uses either comments, questions, familiar topics or routine communication exchanges to support continued interaction. Unlike the other direct assist strategies, topic continuation is most effective when the focus is on increasing the length of the conversation rather than on vocabulary or grammar. The objective is to provide the child with many opportunities to practice conversation while providing the necessary level of modeling and support.

Three different techniques can be used depending on the child and the context, but the goal of each is to maintain active participation in the conversational exchange.

Commenting is the first technique. By following a child's topic initiation with a related comment, s/he is provided with encouragement to explore the topic further, without any direct prompts. Adult attention and added information about the child's topic capitalizes on the shared interest, builds incentive to continue interaction, and reinforces the child's initial conversational interests. Comments can be effective by adding information, modeling related vocabulary and demonstrating continued interest in the current topic.

Questioning is the second technique. It is like commenting in that it signals the child to take a conversational turn and supplies the incentive to continue the interaction. Open-ended questions are most appropriate for extending meaningful conversations, and yes–no questions should be avoided.

Using scripts is the third and most directive type of topic continuation. Scripts utilize a series of repetitive familiar conversational turns that support the interaction because both partners know and fill their prescribed roles. For instance, a greeting routine, daily activity or bedtime ritual can each involve familiar routine communication scripts that are used in the same manner each time the activity is performed. Scripts can be a very effective way of encouraging turn-taking because they do not require children to generate new information but instead leave them free to enjoy the social exchange. Another advantage is that scripted routines encourage the adult to take shorter turns, thus allowing the child more opportunities to practice her/his communication skills.

• *Time delay.* This teaches students to initiate speech in the presence of nonverbal, environmental prompts (Halle *et al.* 1979). The adult targets opportunities to use the time-delay procedure by selecting situations where the child wants access to a desired material or activity and then blocks access to the desired item for a 5–15 second period while maintaining eye contact and an expectant look. If the child responds by correctly labelling the object, the adult provides immediate access to it. If the child does not respond, a corrective prompt or model is provided (see Table 5.3). The most difficult aspect of implementing the time-delay procedure is identifying the appropriate opportunities and implementing the prompting procedures correctly. However, this strategy has been shown to be very effective in teaching students to become less reliant on teachers' verbal prompts and in providing children opportunities to use previously learned language skills (Charlop *et al.* 1985).

• *Incidental teaching.* Unlike the two previous strategies, this relies solely on the child to initiate the teaching interaction and begins with a child requesting an adult's assistance, either verbally or nonverbally. The adult uses this opportunity to require a more complex response from the child. The prompt for a more elaborate communication response can take the form of a request, instruction, model or time-delay, or a combination of these techniques (see Table 5.3).

Conclusion

We know a great deal about effective behavioral strategies for facilitating communication in children with disabilities. Some of our greatest challenges now lie in translating our current knowledge into strategies that are easily used by teachers, caregivers and family members; in developing strategies that are ecologically and socially valid in 'real world' settings (see Brofenbrenner 1979, Schwartz and Baer 1991); and in developing intervention strategies that are culturally responsive and respectful. In this chapter we have attempted to outline some of the major considerations in planning and implementing a behavioral communication intervention. In closing, we would like to summarize the five main points addressed in the chapter.

• Communication is a developmentally important pivotal behavior. Development in other areas is dependent upon and mediated by communication. Delays in communication affect growth in other areas and may be related to challenging behavior. Therefore it is essential to be effective and comprehensive in our intervention efforts.

• Communication is a useful behavior. We need to make sure that interventions focus on form, function and use, and that children learn the power of communication. We need to ensure that interventions result in important and socially valid outcomes for children.

• Communication is a socially based behavior. It is supported by the environment. Children need to have environments that facilitate and support communication and communicative attempts. They also need to be in environments that require (do not preempt) communication and in which there is something to talk about. Children also need to be in environments in which there are interesting communicative partners, both adults and peers.

• Communication is a culturally based behavior. We need to work closely with families to be sure that the communicative interventions are a good match with the family's own communicative styles (*e.g.* language, directiveness, type of technology used).

• Communication is a complex behavior. We need to take a multifaceted approach to assessment and intervention. We need to include a description of the child's strengths and existing supports in the assessment. We also need to make sure that any assessment or intervention strategy is sustainable.

The goal of designing, implementing and evaluating communication interventions is challenging, and it can be extremely rewarding. It is by translating these suggestions into practice—by following the assessment guidelines and selecting from the intervention strategies described above—that interventionists can help children with disabilities become competent in their form, content and use of communication.

REFERENCES

Aram, D., Hall, N. (1989) 'Longitudinal follow-up of children with preschool communication disorders: treatment implications.' *School Psychology Review*, **18**, 487–501.

Bailey, D.B. (1989) 'Case management in early intervention.' *Journal of Early Intervention*, **13**, 120–134.

——McWilliam, R.A. (1990) 'Normalizing early intervention.' *Topics in Early Childhood Special Education*, **10**, 33–47.

—— Wolery, M. (1992) *Teaching Infants and Preschoolers with Disabilities.* New York: Merrill.

Baker, L., Cantwell, P.P. (1982) 'Development, social, and behavioral characteristics of speech and language disorder in children.' *Child Psychiatry and Human Development*, **12**, 195–206.

Bondy A., Frost, L. (1994) *The Picture Exchange Communication System, Training Manual.* Cherry Hill, NJ: Pyramid Educational Consultants.

Bricker, D. (1993) *AEPS Measurement: For Infants and Young Children.* Baltimore: Brookes.

—— (1996) *AEPS Measurement: For Three to Six Years.* Baltimore: Brookes

—— Cripe, J.W. (1992) *An Activity-Based Approach to Early Intervention.* Baltimore: Brookes.

—— Squires, J. (1989) 'The effectiveness of parental screening of at-risk infants: the infant monitoring questionnaires.' *Topics in Early Childhood Special Education*, **9**, 67–85.

Brofenbrenner, U. (1979) *The Ecology of Human Development.* Cambridge, MA: Harvard University Press.

Carr, E.G., Durand, V.M. (1985) 'Reducing behavior problems through functional communication training.' *Journal of Applied Behavior Analysis*, **18**, 111–126.

Charlop, M.H., Schreibman, L., Thibodeau, M.G. (1985) 'Increasing spontaneous verbal responding in autistic children using a time delay procedure.' *Journal of Applied Behavior Analysis*, **18**, 155–166.

Crais, E., Roberts, J.E. (1996) 'Assessing communication skills.' *In:* McLean, M., Bailey, D., Wolery, M. (Eds.) *Assessing Infants And Children With Handicaps.* Columbus, OH: Merrill, pp. 334–397.

Dale, P. (1991) 'The validity of a parent report measure of vocabulary and syntax at 24 months.' *Journal of Speech and Hearing Research*, **34**, 565–571.

Bates, E., Reznick, S., Morisset, C. (1989) 'The validity of a parent report instrument on child language at twenty months.' *Journal of Child Language*, **16**, 239–249.

—— Duchan, J. (1989) 'Evaluating adults' talk to children: assessing adult attunement.' *Seminars in Speech and Language*, **10**, 17–27.

Field, T. (1987) 'Affective and interactive disturbances in infants.' In: Osofsky, J. (Ed.) *Handbook of Infant Development, 2nd Edn.* New York: Wiley, pp. 317–335.

Freeman, S., Dake, L. (1997) *Teach Me Language.* Langley, British Columbia: SKF Books.

Goldstein, H., Hockenberger, E. (1991) 'Significant progress in child language intervention: an 11-year retrospective.' *Research in Developmental Disabilities*, **12**, 401–424.

Guralnick, M.J. (1997) *The Effectiveness of Early Intervention.* Baltimore: Brookes.

Halle, J.W., Marshall, A., Spradlin, J. (1979) 'Time delay: a technique to increase language use and facilitate generalization in retarded children.' *Journal of Applied Behavior Analysis*, **12**, 431–439.

Hart, B.M., Risley, T. (1968) 'Establishing use of descriptive adjectives in the spontaneous speech of disadvantaged preschool children.' *Journal of Applied Behavior Analysis*, **1**, 109–120.

—— —— (1974) 'Using preschool materials to modify the language of disadvantaged children.' *Journal of Applied Behavior Analysis*, **7**, 243–256.

—— —— (1975) 'Incidental teaching of language in the preschool.' *Journal of Applied Behavior Analysis*, **8**, 411–420.

—— —— (1980) 'In vivo language intervention: unanticipated general effects.' *Journal of Applied Behavior Analysis*, **13**, 407–432.

—— —— (1995) *Meaningful Differences in the Everyday Experiences of Young American Children*. Baltimore: Brookes.

Hemmeter, M.L., Kaiser, A.P. (1990) 'Environmental influences on children's language: a model and case study.' *Education and Treatment of Children*, **13**, 331–346.

Hepting, N.H., Goldstein, H. (1996) 'What's natural about naturalistic language intervention?' *Journal of Early Intervention*, **20**, 249–265.

Houghton, J., Bromicki, G., Guess, D. (1987) 'Opportunities to express preferences and make choices among students with severe disabilities in classroom settings.' *Journal of the Association for Persons with Severe Handicaps*, **12**, 18–27.

Kaiser, A.P., Yoder, P.J., Keetz, A. (1992) 'Evaluating milieu teaching.' *In:* Warren, S.F., Reichle, J. (Eds.) *Causes and Effects in Communication and Language Intervention*. Baltimore: Brookes, pp. 9–47.

Klinger, L.G., Dawson, G. (1992) 'Facilitating early social and communicative development in children with autism.' *In:* Warren, S.F., Reichle, J. (Eds.) *Causes and Effects in Communication and Language Intervention*. Baltimore: Brookes, pp. 157–186.

Koegel, L.K. (1995) 'Communication and language intervention.' *In:* Koegel, R.L., Koegel, L.K. (Eds.) *Teaching Children with Autism*. Baltimore: Brookes, pp. 17–32.

—— Koegel, R.K., Dunlap, G. (1996) *Positive Behavioral Support: Including People with Difficult Behavior in the Community*. Baltimore: Brookes.

Koegel, R.L., Frea, W.D. (1993) 'Treatment of social behavior in autism through the modification of pivotal social skills.' *Journal of Applied Behavior Analysis*, **26**, 369–377.

Marfo, K. (1990) 'Maternal directiveness in interactions with mentally handicapped children: an analytical commentary.' *Journal of Child Psychology and Psychiatry*, **31**, 531–549.

McLean, L.K., Cripe, J.W. (1997) 'The effectiveness of early intervention for children with communication disorders.' *In:* Guralnick, M.J. (Ed.) *The Effectiveness of Early Intervention*. Baltimore: Brookes, pp. 349–428.

Moerk, E.L. (1992) *A First Language*. Baltimore: Brookes.

Nye, C., Foster, S., Seaman, D. (1987) 'Effectiveness of language intervention with the language/learning disabled.' *Journal of Speech and Hearing Disorders*, **52**, 348–357.

Olswang, L., Bain, B. (1991) 'Treatment efficacy: when to recommend intervention.' *Language, Speech, and Hearing Services in Schools*, **22**, 255–263.

Ostrosky, M., Kaiser, A. (1991) 'Preschool classroom environments that promote communication.' *Teaching Exceptional Children*, **24** (4), 6–10.

Peck, C. (1985) 'Increasing opportunities for social control by children with autism and severe handicaps.' *Journal of the Association for Persons with Severe Handicaps*, **10**, 183–193.

—— (1989) 'Assessment of social communicative competence: evaluating environments.' *Seminars in Speech and Language*, **10**, 1–15.

Prizant, B., Schuler, A. (1987) 'Facilitating communication: theoretical foundations.' *In:* Cohen, D., Donnellan, A. (Eds.) *Handbook of Autism and Pervasive Developmental Disorders*. New York: Wiley, pp. 289–300.

Rogers-Warren, A.K., Warren, S.F. (1980) 'Mands for verbalizations: facilitating the display of newly trained language in children.' *Behavior Modification*, **4**, 361–382.

—— —— Baer, D.M. (1983) 'Interactional bases of language learning.' *In:* Kernan, K., Begab, M., Edgarton, R. (Eds.) *Environment and Behavior: The Adaptation of Mentally Retarded Persons*. Baltimore: University Park Press, pp. 213–250.

Sainato, D., Carta, J. (1992) 'Classroom influences on the development of social competence in young children with disabilities.' *In:* Odom, S.L., McConnell, S.R., McEvoy, M.A. (Eds.) *Social Competence of Young Children with Disabilities*. Baltimore: Brookes, pp. 93–109.

Schwartz, I.S., Baer, D.M. (1991) 'Social-validity assessments: is current practice state-of-the-art?' *Journal of Applied Behavior Analysis*, **24**, 189–204.

112

—— Olswang, L.B. (1996) 'Documenting child behavior change in naturalistic settings: exploring some data alternatives.' *Topics in Early Childhood Special Education*, **16**, 82–101.

—— Carta, J., McBride, B., Pepler, L. (1993) *Project ECLIPSE Curriculum: Classroom Strategies for Promoting the Communicative Independence of Young Children with Disabilities.* Kansas City: Juniper Gardens Children's Project.

—— —— Grant, S. (1996) 'Examining the use of recommended language intervention practices in early childhood special education classrooms.' *Topics in Early Childhood Special Education*, **16**, 251–272.

Silva, P.A., Williams, S., McGee, R. (1987) 'A longitudinal study of children with developmental language delay at age three: later intelligence, reading, and behavior problems.' *Developmental Medicine and Child Neurology*, **29**, 630–640.

Skinner, B.F. (1957) *Verbal Behavior.* New York: Appleton–Century Crofts.

Tager-Flusberg, H. (1989) 'A pycholinguistic perspective on language development in the autistic child.' *In:* Dawson, G. (Ed.) *Autism: Nature, Diagnosis, and Treatment.* New York: Guilford Press, pp. 92–115.

Theodore, G., Maher, S., Prizant, B. (1990) 'Early assessment and intervention with emotional and behavioral disorders and communication disorders.' *Topics in Language Disorders*, **10**, 42–56.

Walker, D, Greenwood, C., Hart, B., Carta, J., (1994) 'Prediction of school outcomes based on early language production and socioeconomic factors.' *Child Development*, **65**, 606–621.

Warren, S.F., Yoder, P.J. (1994) 'Communication and language intervention: why a constructivist approach is insufficient.' *Journal of Special Education*, **28**, 248–258.

—— Rogers-Warren, A., Baer, D.M., Guess, D. (1980) 'The assessment and facilitation of language generalization.' *In:* Sailor, W., Wilcox, B., Brown, L. (Eds.) *Instructional Design for the Severely Handicapped.* Baltimore: Brookes, pp. 147–181.

Wetherby, A., Prizant, B. (1990) 'Profiling young children's communicative competence.' *In:* Warren & J. Reichle, J. (Eds.) *Causes and Effects in Communication and Language Intervention.* Baltimore: Brookes, pp. 217–253.

6
SENSORY DIFFICULTIES

Maryke Groenveld

Having a new baby can be a scary event, especially if s/he is a first born. Even when the baby arrives into a family with a good support system and is very much wanted, new parenthood is often viewed with some apprehension. Some feel overwhelmed at the prospect of being responsible for the total care and welfare of a completely helpless and dependent being. However, things usually work out much better than expected, and this is by no small means due to the fact that newborns are such excellent teachers. In humans as well as in animals, babies give signals and responses that make the parents touch, nurture and communicate with them. This kind of behavior appears to be largely instinctive on both sides (Stern 1997). What happens, though, when a baby is born blind or deaf? In such cases the bonding process may be impaired or delayed. The parents may feel discouraged by the lack of responsiveness of their baby. They may have the feeling that they are 'not doing it right', which in turn may lead to anxiety and insecurity. This is not necessarily the case for all parents. Unfortunately, few systematic studies are available that have investigated the interactions between deaf or blind parents and their deaf or blind newborns, for it would be interesting to see if they have a different experience. However, this is a rather small group of people, as the majority of deaf or blind children are born to normally hearing or sighted parents.

The way we perceive the world around us, our concept of reality and our relationships with other people are fundamentally embedded in our sensory experiences. Cognitive development is dependent on these experiences and is therefore shaped by the senses (Johnson 1987, Fogel 1997). Thus it stands to reason that the world perception of children with a sensory impairment is different from that of other children and that their development follows a different course (Davidson and Simmons 1992). This does not mean that their world perception is flawed and needs to be reshaped; this premise would not only be arrogant, it would also be impossible. However, children with a sensory impairment live in a world where the majority of people do not experience the world the way they do, and with families who do not share their perceptual experiences. If these children are to be integrated into society, it is important that they learn to share their perceptions with those who experience them in a different way, but without sacrificing their own uniqueness and perceptual integrity. Ideally this process should take the form of mutual habilitation rather than the more one-sided process the term rehabilitation implies. The deaf community is well aware of the need for the preservation of identity and foster a distinct deaf culture. Blind people have also expressed this need (Fogel 1997), but generally do not have as strong a lobby as the deaf community does.

Diagnosis

Children with a visual impairment tend to be diagnosed relatively early in life because most causes are congenital or perinatal (Robinson *et al.* 1987). The condition is usually quite noticeable in children with an ocular disability, but cortical visual impairment is often identified later because the eyes in most cases seem normal (Jan and Groenveld 1993). The diagnosis of children with a congenital hearing impairment is also often late: in a study of 39 cases by Parving (1984), only 33 per cent were diagnosed by the age of 1 year and the parents were usually the initiators of the investigation. Especially if the child is a first born, the parents may not be able to gauge what is normal and may not trust their instinctive feeling that something is not right. It is not uncommon for parents to go to their family doctor and then be told to wait because the child will probably become more responsive with time. Valuable time can be lost this way.

Assessment of development

From an early age, children with a sensory impairment may be subjected to a host of investigations attempting to evaluate their cognitive, linguistic, physical and social development. This is usually not without reason. Parents or caregivers of children with a sensory impairment frequently do not know what to expect, and often progress is not along the predicted lines (Cass *et al.* 1994). These assessments usually involve the use of tests standardized on normally developing children, which consequently do not take into account the unique developmental patterns of children with sensory impairment. This has often led to discussing development in terms of delay rather than acknowledging developmental differences. The nature of these differences is difficult to gauge as well, especially with the blind. Blindness is a rare condition, total blindness even more so. Especially in countries where there are no, or limited, residential education facilities for the blind, study populations tend to be small, which makes generalization more difficult. Blindness also rarely occurs in isolation. It is therefore not unlikely that research involving blind children deals with effects that may be partly due to other, coexisting conditions or at least to an interaction with these conditions. Studies of children with retinopathy of prematurity (ROP) are a case in point. There is a considerable amount of information on the development of preterm children with a very low birthweight (Saigal *et al.* 1990, Hack *et al.* 1992). Often studies of totally blind children involve a number of children with ROP, yet when these groups of children are compared with normally sighted children, all the effects are usually attributed to the blindness.

Testing the deaf with standardized material is also fraught with difficulty, especially where the language component is concerned. If the child is using sign language, all verbal components of the test need to be translated into sign, which invalidates the standardization. It becomes even more complicated if the assessment has to be done with the aid of an interpreter, for not only is the standardization of the test material jeopardized, but also the examiner may not know what the interpreter and the child are saying. This is not so much of a problem with a well-trained, professional interpreter, but these are not always available. Sometimes the signing skills of the child surpass those of the interpreter and the finer nuances of the responses are lost. Occasionally a parent acts as an interpreter and may be inclined to communicate what they know their child knows, rather than what the child actually signs.

CASE STUDY
Debbie came to the assessment with her interpreter, who had known her for a long time. The interpreter was asked to stay as close as she could to what was said, while she was signing. She also was asked to speak what she was signing so that the examiner would have a better understanding of the content of the conversation. However, the interpreter declined because she felt it would interfere with the spontaneity of the conversation. Since the examiner understood some sign, she was still able to read some of what was communicated. For the question, "What is the color of grass?" the interpreter signed: grass, what color, red or green? When the examiner was asked not to give examples, because this would change the value of the answers, the interpreter answered: that would not be fair, that way she would never get it right.

Testing a hearing impaired child who is trained to communicate with an oral method poses the same problems as testing a visually impaired child: we do not really know which normative group to compare the child to, or what the test findings mean. When we find a language delay in a hearing impaired child or a visual perceptual delay in a visually impaired child, are these delays related to the sensory impairment or are there other underlying causes? It would be erroneous to assume that cognitive difficulties of a child with a sensory impairment are always due to that impairment and that the children in question are not subject to learning disabilities as well, especially when one takes into account that sensory impairments often do not come alone. The problem is not so much with obtaining accurate test data, but rather with how to interpret them, especially when the impairment is partial. Even when the impairment is total, the test results obtained through the intact sense are not directly comparable to those of a child without such an impairment (Groenveld 1990, Netelenbos and Savelsbergh 1991).

Interpretations of test scores would be easier if they were absolute markers of what a child is capable of doing, but unfortunately most tests, especially those of cognitive function, provide a comparison with a normative group on a rather arbitrarily chosen set of tasks. Tests have been developed that have been standardized for children with a specific sensory impairment, but these do not always provide enough information when decisions have to be made with regard to the child's ability to participate in an integrated setting, where the child may be the only one with the sensory impairment, nor are they always suitable for children with a partial impairment. Some evaluators have opted for omitting those parts of tests which would put children with a sensory impairment at an unfair disadvantage, but this practice has the problem of extrapolating information from one area of cognitive function to others which have never been measured (Groenveld 1990). This does not mean that assessment information on children with a sensory impairment is without value, but it needs to be stressed that it should always be paired with direct observation and validated with the help of people who know the children well, *e.g.* parents, caregivers and teachers. Group testing should not be considered. The predictive value of the assessment should be treated with caution as well: the predictive value of test results will be greatly reduced if there is a significant difference in experience between the child being tested and the normative group (Salvia and Ysseldyke 1981). As with any child, the progress of a child with a sensory impairment should be monitored in the light of new experiences and opportunities rather than with set expectations. Since a sensory impairment will affect all aspects of the child's development, a multidisciplinary assessment across a range of naturalistic settings will yield the most useful information. The team members should be thoroughly familiar with the effects of the sensory impairment, and the parents or caregivers should play an integral role. This will allow for validation of the information across disciplines and settings, and ensures that the information can be used as the basis for intervention. Appointing a case manager will make transfer of information to the community easier as well as providing a liaison when changes in circumstances necessitate a new evaluation. When there is no other option than to have the child assessed by individual professionals, it will be very important that these people are experienced with the particular sensory impairment.

Parental reaction to diagnosis of sensory impairment

When parents are confronted with the diagnosis of sensory impairment, their first reaction is often one of shock and disbelief, then followed by grief. If this grieving process is prolonged, or unacknowledged, or if the parents are not receiving adequate support, it may affect the relationship between the parents and the child (Sloman *et al.* 1993). This does not only happen with newborns.

CASE STUDY
Jamie had become totally blind due to retinal detachment after years of partial sight. The effect on the family was devastating. His parents, especially his mother, were depressed for a long time. Jamie became much more fearful and clingy than he had been before, and during the office visits both he and his mother would be crying to the point that it was very difficult to carry out an assessment of any kind. The family were given support services, but the bulk of them were directed to Jamie or dealt mainly with factual information for the parents, rather than addressing their emotional needs. In a follow-up evaluation several years later Jamie seemed to have adjusted well to his blindness. He was outgoing and communicative, had friends in school, and had made good academic progress. To him his blindness seemed more an attribute than a burden. His mother, however, had not fared as well. She still appeared depressed, cried when she reported on his progress, and still actively mourned the fact that he was different from other children. She felt guilty that she could not have presented her husband with a 'better child'. Jamie was worried about the fact that his mother was always sad about him and that he could not make her happy regardless of what he did. When he was asked to make three wishes, they centered around his mother rather than himself.

Although resources had been put in place for Jamie, and his parents had been given a lot of information, they had not worked through the grieving process and ultimately did not accept Jamie for what he now was: a successful blind child rather than a failed sighted child. In spite of this Jamie was fortunate in that he had the support services he needed.

Sometimes the parents' grief and denial keeps them from using the available services or from making critical decisions. This can have serious consequences. In newborns the areas in the brain that process sensory information are not fully developed and depend on specific sensory stimulation to mature. If this input is not forthcoming the centers originally designated to process this information may lose the capability to do so (Fish 1983, Kalil 1987). It is therefore important that parents are given ample access to professional support.

Support for parents

Having to adjust to the realization that their child has a sensory impairment, as well as having to care for an infant with special needs and often for a young family as well, can be quite a burden. Thus, when the diagnosis is made, the parents should be connected with a multi-disciplinary support team. This team will need to provide them not only with the factual information they need with regard to the sensory disability, but also with support to help them adapt to this. Again, parents should be an integral part of this team and be made to feel that they are in control. Appointing a case manager to coordinate the services will ensure greater continuity and will make it much easier for the parents to secure access to help when they need it (Youngson-Reilly *et al.* 1994). Ongoing assistance in practical interactive skills with a sensory impaired child is essential. This does not mean that parents should constantly be confronted by teams of experts: this could seriously interfere with their natural parenting skills and turn the child into some kind of communal project. Sensitive, integrated support of the budding relationship between the parent and the infant, which will point them in the direction of greater opportunity for interaction and exploration, is of the essence. It is important for parents to know that there is someone they can talk to when they need practical information or when they feel overwhelmed by unexpected demands. Bringing parents of recently diagnosed children into contact with experienced parents of children with a similar condition is also often perceived as helpful and supportive.

Several studies have assessed stress levels in parents of children with sensory disabilities. Mothers generally reported higher stress levels than fathers (Meadow-Orlans *et al.* 1995). Parents with less education tended to report higher stress levels than those with more education (Brand and Coetzer 1994). This would suggest that proper support is essential and that the level of complexity of the information should be matched to the people it serves. Quite often parents with limited reading skills are provided with sophisticated articles or books which go well beyond their reading levels. Frequently the amount of background information they would need to understand the material is lacking. Direct contact with people who can translate professional information in understandable lay terms may be more helpful. Not infrequently, parents of newly diagnosed children complain that their ophthalmologist or otolaryngologist did not tell them anything, while the specialist concerned felt that a considerable amount of time had been spent carefully explaining the condition. Sometimes both parties do not seem to speak the same language, and when someone does not understand what it is they don't understand, it can become very difficult to ask questions. Konstantareas and Lampropoulou (1995) found that low self-esteem was the best predictor of high stress levels in mothers. This emphasizes the importance of ensuring that the parents feel empowered by the support services, rather than being left with the feeling that their abilities are limited, and that they know there is someone to take over when the difficulties become too overwhelming.

Interventions to promote optimum development

ENCOURAGING EXPLORATION OF THE ENVIRONMENT

Since the brain of an infant depends on stimulation for its development, the importance of early intervention cannot be emphasized enough. However, not all stimulation necessarily promotes brain development. Some people have the mistaken belief that if children have reduced vision, they need to be surrounded by auditory stimulation. They may provide the child with a wide array of noisy toys over which s/he has little control, and leave the radio on all day. Rather than stimulating awareness of sound, this can have the opposite effect. The child may learn to suppress all this noise, become less alert to environmental sound, and thus have a reduced opportunity to discover the meaning of the sound. Helping the child in a meaningful way to explore the relationship between sound and the object or person that produces it will provide much more information than random noise.

For visually impaired children, the particular diagnosis can have immediate implications for intervention. For instance, if the child has a visual impairment that is associated with a high degree of light sensitivity, then reduction of light levels and avoidance of bright lights may have a positive effect on the amount and frequency of visual stimulation. Several countries now have vision stimulation teachers who get involved with children from a very early age. They can assist the parents with implementing activity programs which not only promote the use of residual visual skills, but also employ methods and suggestions that help the child explore the environment more actively. Children with very limited vision are often not aware of objects around them and are therefore not as likely to reach out for and explore them. As this also tends to keep them out of trouble it may not be immediately identified as a problem. Some blind babies may be too 'good' and lie in their cribs for hours on end without disturbing anybody. Although tired parents may not complain, this is not necessarily a good thing. During these passive periods very little exploration goes on and therefore very few new skills are learned. Even their muscle tone is often lower. Most young children with a severe visual impairment have residual vision, but they may be able to see only objects that are close to their body, and therefore they are not as likely to try to move to get them. Tying a string to an interesting toy, preferably one that can move and produces sound, and then very slowly pulling the toy in a direction *away* from the child, may entice the child to follow. This way children can be encouraged to move of their own free will, and if other interesting objects are positioned along the way, they may become aware that there are things out there to be explored, but that you have to move to find them.

Anyone who has been around typical infants realizes that communication and exploration of cause and effect goes on a long time before the child has distinct words. Before they develop language, normally sighted children can indicate an interest by looking at an object. By looking at what the child is looking at, the parent can comment on it, provide the object and encourage exploration. The blind child cannot indicate an interest in this way and therefore may have less opportunity to initiate interactions and explorations. Moreover, since they do not have as many opportunities to observe cause and effect simultaneously the way normally sighted children do, their understanding of such connections may be delayed.

Blind infants are much more dependent on touch and hearing than sighted children for gathering information about the world around them. This relates to touching as well as being touched. Fogel (1997) suggests that continuous, mutual interpersonal touching could serve the same role as visual contact does for sighted children in the process of communication, because the child would be more aware of the continuous presence of the communication partner. Helping parents of blind babies become more comfortable with their own and their child's bodies may create more spontaneous touching and thus provide a climate that is more conducive to communication (Franco *et al.* 1996).

UNDERSTANDING OBJECT RELATIONSHIPS

Preisler (1995) conducted an interesting longitudinal study comparing the development of communication in blind infants and deaf infants. She concentrated on preverbal abilities, exploration of toys, social and symbolic play, communicative intent and sharing experiences. Compared to deaf infants, blind infants were more delayed in their development of communication; the author points out that in infancy, visual stimulation may play a more critical role than auditory stimulation. The deaf child has the advantage of being able to indicate a shared interest by directed gaze and by being able to observe reciprocal play. Sharing and turn taking are essential elements in communication. These elements may be much more difficult to model when a child is blind. With partially sighted children it is very important that the person communicating with the child comes close enough to be observed.

Early exploration is also more difficult for a blind child: vision allows us to observe objects, aspects of objects and their relationship to other objects simultaneously. Thus, the sensory experience is much more immediate. Even when the child is not actively playing with the object it is still there and demonstrates its presence by being in the child's line of vision. Auditory information is sequential, it is there and then it is gone. If a deaf infant plays with a toy and drops it, the toy will still be present, provided the child saw it fall. For blind children, the object will be gone when it is dropped, because for them the sound the object makes when it falls is not necessarily related to the object itself. Sound and object may both be registered, but the connection may not be made. Therefore for the blind child, interest in the object may be lost earlier than for the deaf child. This in turn could lead to less time spent in active exploration, resulting in less information that can be shared. When blind infants are playing, it may be helpful to have them play with objects on a tray with a rim around it so that they are not so easily pushed out of reach. Toys that make a sound when they are moved can also provide more information about their location: when they fall or roll away, the sound made will be more closely related to the sounds encountered by children during active play. This may give them a greater opportunity to discover that the toy is still close by, although they can no longer touch it.

For a deaf child the world is centered in the reach of the eyes. What is not within the visual field is not there, and just as blind children need to learn to search, so may the deaf need to learn to scan. Netelenbos and Savelsbergh (1991) found that deaf children, even as late as the early teens, were less able than sighted children to catch a ball which came from outside the visual field, although there was no such difference when the ball came from inside the visual field. They suggested that a lack of auditory stimulation during development can lead to deficiencies in the coordination of actions, such as catching, which are both spatially and temporally constrained. Although deaf children are able to observe objects and relationships between them, as well as to watch people and their body language, it may be much more difficult to connect present experiences with previous ones, if they do not have sufficient language to connect them. Similarly, it will be harder for the people around them to alert them to the similarities and differences if they do not have sufficient shared language to do so. Some deaf children may therefore live more in the present because their more limited language and verbal reasoning skills may make it more difficult for them to learn from past complex experiences and to extrapolate to the future. In this respect some of them may resemble children with attention deficit disorder, although they may not share the condition.

For both deaf and blind children, tasks such as categorizing and generalizing may cause difficulty. Blind children do not see the objects in their natural groupings or functions and therefore may not always develop the prelingual concept of the group that is later matched with a word. This is not to say that they that they will not use the category word, but they may attach a different meaning to it and thus it is more difficult to share with others. Deaf children will have access to the visual information but may not have the language to describe the connections with other observations to themselves. This may be one of the reasons why deaf children of deaf parents do better: they have a consistent shared language system which allows them to make the connections consistently, rather than intermittently, as is the case with a deaf child in an environment where only a few people sign or where very little of the spoken language is understood. Both groups, as well as children with a partial impairment, could benefit from activities around the house which involve sorting: putting cutlery away, forks with forks, spoons with spoons, etc., as well as placing all the cutlery in the drawer, all the pots on the shelf and so on. In this way they get an opportunity to realize that objects can be ordered in many different ways. Later this can be expanded to more abstract categories such as sensory properties, emotions, etc. These kinds of domestic activities have the added advantage that they can be shared in a natural environment. The parent is not the teacher, rather the child is the helper. This is especially important since most children with a sensory impairment are already subjected to a much greater amount of deliberate teaching at an early age than other children. This can result in a diminished need for independent exploration that is not directly an effect of the impairment. Early intervention needs to have a fine balance between avoidance of understimulation and respect for independent, spontaneous exploration.

THE USE OF TOYS

In play, the use of household objects may provide a greater amount of information than most commonly available toys. A large number of preschool toys are based on a visual similarity with common objects, which may be difficult to appreciate for a child with a visual impairment. Many are made of the same kind of material (plastic) and differ little from each other in taste, smell or tactile quality. Using, for instance, an orange instead of a plastic ball to encourage the child to roll an object back and forth, or using a metal pot and a wooden spoon rather than a plastic drum, may encourage the children to stay longer with the objects because there is more to explore, while they are exposed to the same abstract concepts, such as shape, size, cause and effect, etc. Many young children without a sensory impairment also seem to prefer real things. Often parents have assigned their toddlers a kitchen cupboard in which they are allowed free reign (and have the dented pot lids to show for it). Many young children on Christmas morning play more happily with the boxes than with the toys. When professionals try to determine whether an environment is properly stimulating for a young child, it may be wiser to assess what kind of experiences the child has during the course of a day rather than how many toys are present.

INCREASING SOCIAL INTERACTIONS

Many children with a sensory impairment have limited opportunity for social interactions, for a variety of reasons. Not only do they often lack a shared reference base, which makes it difficult for them to enter the play of children whose experiences are different from their own, but also they are frequently surrounded by adults. This makes it even more difficult for them to experiment with approach strategies, and it inhibits other children from approaching them. Parents of children with a sensory impairment often complain that their children do not have close friends and are never invited to 'sleep-overs' or birthday parties. Preisler (1997) notes that although a great deal of energy is put into teaching blind children concrete skills, such as developing better gross and fine motor skills, or teaching language through object identification, very little attention is payed to discussing feelings, humour and a sense of belonging. Conversations between parents and blind children tend to be much more directive and include less about the experience of emotions. Preisler points out that it must be difficult for blind children to form an inner representation of other people whom they cannot see, and who do not make themselves known to them. She considers that in this respect deaf children have a greater opportunity to take part in the external world. However, although deaf children may have more opportunity to participate in the here and now, for them it may be much more difficult to relate current experiences to others through language.

For parents there is often the more immediate concern of how to bring their children into contact with others. A tempting home environment can be a first step. If there are interesting things for other children to do, they may be more willing to overcome their fear of the unknown and play with a child who may not always react in an accustomed manner. For example, a jungle gym in the garden, or a pizza party in the kitchen where the children can make their own pizzas with some help, could provide powerful incentives and a good opportunity to learn how to share. When there are concrete things to do, the focus is not on the social contact alone, and this will make it easier for the sensory impaired child to enter the play situation. It is usually better to keep the duration of the contacts short, especially initially, and to end the visit before there are altercations. If the children are still young, it will be a good idea to invite mothers along, so that the visiting child has a familiar person around. It also helps the mother of the typical child to overcome her apprehension about how to communicate with and what to expect of a child with a severe sensory impairment, thereby increasing the likelihood of a reciprocal invitation. Even if initially the play is completely parallel, this should not discourage the parent of the sensory impaired child, as interactive play skills are not learned in one session. Inviting only one other child at a time avoids the typically developing children playing with each other to the exclusion of the child with the sensory impairment. Sharing transportation to and from school can also be a way to bring an isolated child into contact with her/his peers. Of course, these activities are much harder to arrange for parents who work, but it that case some shared activities for the children can be planned for the weekend.

When the child with a sensory impairment begins to become aware that s/he is 'different' it is important to encourage contacts with children who share their perceptual differences. Especially for older children in integrated schools, camps for the hearing or visually impaired can be powerful experiences. In these settings they are no longer unique and they have opportunities to experience their strengths in ways that are not easily accommodated in an integrated setting. Although there are residential schools for the deaf in British Columbia, where this author is from, there are no longer any residential schools for the blind. During a visit to such a school in England, it was a revelation to see the natural leadership qualities some of the children there had developed, and the ability of these children to take care of peers whom they perceived as being in greater need of protection. Because they were less isolated, many seemed to have developed a stronger self-concept. This does not mean to say that children in integrated settings cannot develop a positive self-concept, but this may need to be much more carefully fostered to avoid it being extinguished by a mistaken perception of helplessness by those around them. Creating interesting environments where children with a sensory impairment can explore safely can also have a broadening effect. Unfortunately this is easier said than done: the incidence of sensory impairment is low, and often the expense involved in creating these environments cannot be justified by the local education authorities.

CHOOSING A MODE OF COMMUNICATION FOR DEAF CHILDREN

Many parents of children with sensory impairments have to make critical decisions, often fairly soon after the diagnosis has been made. In particular, the parents of deaf children are faced with a very early dilemma: should their child be raised with sign language, total communication or auditory/oral communication, and furthermore, should the possibility of a cochlear implant be explored? It is often difficult for such parents to obtain unbiased information, since all camps seem to have staunch supporters and antagonists. All modes of communication have advantages and disadvantages. Children who sign have a complete language at their disposal, with its own grammar and idiom. However, if they live in an environment where few other people sign, they still can be very isolated and limited in their opportunity to develop their language skills fully. It is not unusual that in a family only the mother of the deaf child gets actively involved in sign language. The deaf child is then not only isolated from the community, but also from the rest of the family. This has social as well as cognitive implications. Some Deaf activists, at least in North America, have gone as far as stating that deaf children are *de facto* members of the Deaf community and that if they are born to hearing parents, which is the case for more than 90 per cent of deaf children, they should be turned over to the Deaf community to be acculturated (Balkany *et al.* 1996). This process is referred to as horizontal acculturation, as opposed to vertical acculturation whereby cultural values are transmitted from one generation to another within family structures. This would mean removing the child from the home into a residential Deaf school (Lane 1993), where the Deaf community takes on the responsibility for determining and teaching the value patterns. The crucial part in this is not whether a young child should be in a residential school or not, but who should make the decision, the parents or the Deaf community, and who is responsible for the transmission of the belief systems. For some children there is no other option than a residential school if they want to become fluent communicators in sign language, especially if they live far away from resources. However, ultimately it should be the parents who make these decisions, because, as Balkany *et al.* (1996) state, they care more deeply for their child, know their child best and are involved in all aspects of the child's life. It is not that long ago that massive horizontal acculturation programs were carried out with large numbers of North American and Australian First Nations people, often with disastrous results.

Cochlear implants are another option. They consist of a device, part of which is surgically implanted, that can provide sound information to some of those who do not benefit from traditional hearing or vibrotactile aids. They are used in children with congenital deafness as well as children with acquired profound hearing loss. A position paper by the Canadian Association of Speech–Language Pathologists and Audiologists (Durieux-Smith *et al.* 1995) summarized that children with profound postlingual deafness benefit from multichannel cochlear implants in a way similar to postlingually deafened adults. In children with pre-lingual deafness the gains are more gradual, and although improvements do occur with time, there is considerable variability. The age of the child at the time of the implantation is a factor, and several studies have advocated implantation as early as possible (*e.g.* Miyamoto *et al.* 1997, Tyler *et al.* 1997), since early implants seemed to correspond with greater gains. Ponton *et al.* (1996) have shown that maturation of cortical auditory function does not progress during deafness, but that most, although not all of the maturational processes resume after implantation in children. Some activists in the (American) Deaf community have been very resistant to such implants. They maintain that deafness is not an illness that needs to be cured (Swanson 1997), and that implants remove the children from the minority cultural entity to which they belong; even terms such as genocide have been used. This has made it rather difficult for parents of deaf children to obtain unbiased information. Some children with implants in schools for the deaf feel discriminated against and stop using their devices. Balkany *et al.* (1996) report that the new sign in American Sign Language for a cochlear implant is the same as for a snake bite behind the ear. This lack of acceptance may be a factor behind the study reported by Rose *et al.* (1996). They studied 151 prelingually deaf children with implants in schools for the deaf and reported that 47 per cent were no longer wearing the implant. In the remaining 53 per cent they were unable to determine who was deriving benefit from the device but stated that many indicated despondency over the results of the implant. When parents decide to opt for a cochlear implant they also need to make sure that appropriate training and support for using the device is available and whether or nor educational changes need to be made.

With the oral-only approach, children are given early amplification of their residual hearing and are taught listening and lip-reading skills. This method is not without its problems either. The approach frequently implies a promise of full integration in the hearing world, provided the parents follow the correct procedure. However, many children with severe or profound hearing loss do not become fully integrated in the hearing world and continue to have difficulty communicating, although the parents may have done exactly what they were supposed to do. Parents may end up blaming themselves for the lack of success, not realizing that the promises were unrealistic to begin with. Another problem with the oral-only approach is exclusion of sign, finger spelling and gesture, because this is felt to be interfering with the development of good listening skills and speech. This assumption has never been formally put to the test, and it may remove important clues to information that was not properly heard or understood. Many cultures have an elaborate system of signs and gestures that are used in combination with the oral language and add to the meaning and emotional tone of the conversation. Although these gestures are not necessarily formally taught, they seem to follow specific patterns that are quite clear to those familiar with the language, but not necessarily to outsiders. Even blind children use gestures, and they resemble those of sighted children both in form and content. Iverson and Goldin-Meadow (1997) have suggested that gesture also serves a function for the speaker, independent of the effect on the listener.

Proponents of total communication advocate a system whereby the child uses whatever means are available and suitable to develop and maintain early communication (Freeman *et al.* 1981). The method combines amplification, sign language, finger spelling and auditory/oral methods. The primary interest of this method is in the result (functional communication skills) rather than the method by which it is obtained. Of course proponents of the other methods will proclaim that this is their goal as well, but the total communication method seems to pay greater heed to the natural communication style of the individual child.

Since the field appears to be so polarized, it may be difficult for the parents of deaf children to obtain unbiased information about the optimal communication method for their child. Whichever method they choose will involve a lot of effort and commitment on their part as well as on the child's and will have a profound effect on the child's life. It would therefore seem more just if the children themselves could be involved in the choice of method. Indeed, some Deaf activists have proposed that parents delay the decision about a cochlear implant until the children are old enough to decide for themselves. However, by that time the opportunity to make full use of the implant will be lost, since the critical time for starting to use hearing and speech may be over and the cortical potential may no longer be there (Cohen 1994, Balkany *et al.* 1996).

It will be important for the parents to visit several different programs before they make their choice. It is also helpful to get in touch with other parents of older deaf children to see how they arrived at their decision and how they communicate now. Getting in contact with deaf adults may help to modify some preconceived ideas about deafness, as well as adding a longer term perspective to the decision. When this is done, it should be kept in mind that these meetings will always be with individual people, not with representatives of a particular communication method, and that the experiences of the people the parents meet will not necessarily be those of their own child. When a communication mode is chosen that involves sign language it is very important that the whole family participates, as well as significant people outside the family.

Although their sensory impairments are quite different, blind and deaf children both show delayed and unusual patterns of language development. Interestingly, among hearing impaired children, deaf children of deaf parents seem to do the best, although their numbers are very small. Prendergast and McCollum (1996) found that deaf mothers and deaf toddlers tended to be much more attentive to communication with each other than toddlers and their

125

hearing mothers. Schilling and DeJesus (1993) reported that deaf children with deaf mothers appeared to experience fewer problems not just in language acquisition but in other areas of development too. This may be related to the fact that these children are culturally better integrated in their environment and therefore are exposed to information and experiences with greater consistency. They also are likely to be more accepted socially and emotionally. It is unlikely that deaf parents will grieve when they realize that their child is deaf. It would be interesting to see if there are parallels among blind children born to blind parents.

LANGUAGE DEVELOPMENT IN CHILDREN WITH VISUAL IMPAIRMENT

It is difficult to understand how language develops in the absence of vision, since so much of early learning seems to be based on visual input. However, some researchers have questioned how large a role vision actually plays (Landau 1997, Locke 1997). They point out that blind children do not seem to have difficulty with learning to speak in meaningful sentences. They propose that the capacity to do so is genetically determined. However, producing a sentence that is a meaningful unit on its own is not necessarily the same as forming a sentence that refers to a shared experience and is used in a meaningful exchange of information. Congenitally blind children are frequently quite capable of producing grammatically impressive sentences that seem to have little connection with the situation at hand. This ability is often mistaken for conversational expertise. Moreover, since children with congenital blindness tend to spend much of their time with adults, they tend to pattern their speech on adult models, which can make it even more difficult for them to interact with other children. Some of the children in the clinic with which this author has been involved would progress from complete sentences that were only very marginally related to the topic of conversation to more telegraphic speech, conveying more information. Although in sentence structure this would seem to be a regression, in functional communication it was a gain. McConachie (1990) found that it seemed to be especially the totally blind who tended to use expressive language that was beyond their level of comprehension, while severely visually impaired children who used visually directed reaching did not. However, this was not the case for all totally blind children; for many their expressive language was behind their level of comprehension, with first words sometimes not emerging until 2 years of age. None of the children in the study were reported to have other disabilities. Perez-Pereira (1994), in a single-case study of twins where one was blind and the other not, found that the blind girl was much more inclined to use imitations, repetitions and routines in her speech than her sighted sister. By varying some elements or expanding the information, the blind girl learned to use her language in a more pragmatic way. Gaines and Halpern-Felsher (1995) conducted a similar study with deaf twins who were both enrolled in a total communication preschool. Again, the hearing twin's communications tended to be more responsive, while the deaf twin tended to use more imitative signs and gestures.

INCREASING SOCIAL PLAY

When children with a profound hearing or visual impairment enter preschool or daycare they are often isolated and demonstrate poor play skills. Teachers frequently have little or no experience of the impairment and may not understand the child's unique development.

In countries where infant services for sensory impaired children are available it is found to be helpful if the staff are prepared for the child's arrival by the parents as well as by the infant worker. The child can be prepared for the transition by a couple of visits with a familiar adult. This is not only helpful in the preschool years, but also later. Especially for blind students it is important to have a number of orientation and mobility sessions in the new facility before the transition is made.

Preisler (1993) reported from her longitudinal study that blind children's behavior in preschool is often quite different from that of sighted children. She found that blind children rarely entered sighted child's play and rarely initiated contact. The sighted children initially expressed an interest in the blind child, but since this was not reciprocated their attention quickly faded. This may not always be because the blind child lacks play entry skills, but sometimes because the signals for a request for entry and an invitation to join are not mutually recognized or cannot be interpreted in a meaningful way.

CASE STUDY
Tanya is a bright 4-year-old who has been totally blind since birth. It was her first day in her new preschool. Soon she attracted the interest of Jenny, an equally bright 4-year-old, who wanted to play with her. In the usual fashion that children initiate play contact, Jenny started to play beside Tanya with a box of large cards and was soon joined by two other (sighted) girls. Tanya, who was no fool, also seemed to know the rules: you don't ask if you can play, you start to do the same thing. First she made a number of unintelligible sounds, which resembled the environmental sounds, but contained no meaning for the other girls, because they were not attuned to them. So she reached for where the sound had come from, found a card and started to fan herself with it. This was apparently not what she was supposed to do and her actions drew some telling looks from the other children, which Tanya obviously missed and therefore did not adapt her behavior. The play did not progress much, nor was it particularly interesting to either party, so Tanya tried to pick up on other clues. She heard someone say the word mess, a term she was quite familiar with. She then tried to enter the play verbally and said: "You are making a mess, you guys, put it where it belongs, you are making a mess." This drew surprised looks from the other girls, because the original remark had come from another group behind them and they had not payed attention to it. But Jenny, who was willing to give it a try, said: "Yes, don't be messy", thus making an attempt to follow Tanya's lead. But since there was no mess and no other activity had been initiated, the interaction came to a standstill again. Tanya, who was used to filling awkward pauses with polite conversation, because she had often heard it around her, said to the air in front of her: "What is your name?" Jenny, who realized that this question was probably directed to her, told Tanya, but did not ask for hers, since the teacher had told her already. Tanya then quickly followed up by asking if she had any brothers or sisters and asked for their names and age, height, grade in school, and so on. Jenny, who could not see why all this information was important to Tanya, decided to move to a topic that interested her and Tanya was sure to know a lot about. She turned to Tanya and said: "You are blind, right? People who can't see are called blinded"—thereby picking the only topic Tanya knew absolutely nothing about because she had no concept of sight. She said "Yes" in a rather confused tone and started fanning herself with the card. At this point both gave up on the conversation. Jenny now also picked up a card and started fanning herself, thus again trying to enter Tanya's play, an activity that was lost on Tanya.

On the surface, Tanya's behavior looked odd and poorly adapted, and indeed she ended up alone as the other three girls gave up and found something else to do. However, this was not because proper procedures had not been followed. Both girls had tried to enter the other's play by starting parallel play, but their perceptions of the cues were so different that they could not be shared. An intervenor could have tried to set up a situation where the opportunities for shared experience and references were greater. This does not mean that adults should always act as mediators between the sensory impaired child and typically developing peers. In this way important initiation skills are either not learned or not practised, which can lead to further isolation. Rather, the intervenor could create a situation that both children can recognize more readily and where there is a better chance for both to enter each other's play. This problem of isolation within a peer group is not exclusive to blind children: hearing impaired children in integrated settings frequently communicate only with their interpreter (Shaw and Jamieson 1997), and in this way the intervenor can become a barrier between the child and the social environment rather than an aide.

NATURALISTIC TEACHING

The need for experiences in their natural settings and sequences cannot be stressed enough for both hearing impaired and visually impaired children. Both have difficulty in acquiring concepts that can be readily shared with those who acquire their concepts through different means. Although we happily teach children all kinds of things, we do not really know how they learn. Somehow, without being specifically taught, they eventually learn that a poodle and a boxer are both dogs and a sheep is not, in spite of the considerable similarities between sheep and poodles. The ability is probably developed through awareness of a host of information that is assimilated without being consciously pointed out. If we start to teach children with a sensory impairment concepts outside of their natural setting, we start making assumptions about which are the critical attributes and which are not. Unfortunately, we do not know exactly what these critical attributes are. If we leave the concept to be taught within the natural sequence and setting, then the incidental information will remain intact and can be better assimilated by the child. This may then give the child the opportunity to correct for any faulty assumptions we may make about how they acquire new concepts. In addition, the expectation a person has about what s/he is about to hear or see in a given situation may affect the perceptual organization of what s/he is attending to, especially if that information is ambiguous. Children with a sensory impairment are likely to be able to use their residual sensory ability more effectively if the objects or concepts they are expected to perceive belong in the setting in which they are presented. The likelihood of visual recognition of a spoon or a plate during dinnertime is much higher than when it is pulled out of the teacher's bag during 'visual stimulation time'. Creating natural settings for visual and auditory recognition can be a powerful aid in stimulating the use of residual vision or hearing. Effective teaching is also more likely to occur in situations that occur at regular intervals during the day, such as mealtimes, bathtime, etc. They also offer a better opportunity for spontaneous, unintentional practice. Body parts and their relative positions are much more easily taught in the bathroom, with more opportunity for exploration and repetition, than in the classroom. This does not mean that natural settings for teaching cannot be created in school situations as well. The critical part is that the experience is used to teach language rather than using language to refer to an implied experience. Natural settings also create a greater opportunity for a shared focus, which reduces the likelihood of faulty feedback. When a hearing impaired child makes an approximation to a word and the hearing person does not quite understand, usually a repetition is asked for. If that still does not result in clarity, the hearing person often makes an educated guess at what the child is trying to talk about and bases the response on that assumption. If the child was trying to say something else, the feedback does not support the original statement and confusion ensues. Blind children who use more holistic patterns may produce sentences where some of the words are related to the topic of the conversation but not to the meaning of the sentence itself. The listener may then respond to the content of the sentence rather than the intent, and this could result in an unintended shift of topic. A natural setting in both cases would offer greater opportunity to refocus on a common topic and offer tangible support for the intended communication.

CASE STUDY
Paul is a 6-year-old boy who was totally blind from birth. He was quite isolated in his class and spent most of his time with his teacher's aide. Since finger painting was on the curriculum and the incentive was to normalize Paul as much as possible, he participated in finger painting as well, together with his aide, who verbalized for him what he was doing. She told him where the individual pots with color were in front of him and asked him to select particular colors. She commented on how pretty his picture was and encouraged him to go all the way to the edges of his paper. Paul answered all his aide's questions about what he was painting, what his favorite color was and asked her if he should add a little more pink or not.

Although Paul was being taught a number of useful skills during this activity, such as spatial awareness in trying to go to the edge of the paper and localization in trying to find particular paint pots, he also was performing a number of actions that made little sense to him. Although it is of some value for a blind child to know that grass is green, because that is a common base of reference and when the grass is yellow it may need water, it is of little interest to him whether he uses green or pink paint, nor does what he paints make any sense to him. This activity could equally well be carried out with elements that had more meaning for him. Since he was socially quite isolated, the training of spatial awareness could have included other children as well. Instead of three pots of paint, Paul could have been provided with jars with jam, honey and peanut butter. He also could have been given bread, crackers and cookies. Other children could have come to his store and taken turns to place their orders. Paul could have used smell to identify the toppings and touch to find the proper base, and used a knife to spread each topping to the edges. After having done this for a while, he could have taken his place in line and placed his order just like the others. To ensure that this procedure went smoothly, he could have practised it first with his aide. For art activities, more tactile media such as clay or playdough will offer much more opportunity for artistic expression in blind children than paints or markers. Deaf children could participate in the store activity in a similar way. The activity can be expanded by grouping sweet and savory toppings together, as well as soft and brittle bases. The opportunities for variation are endless and the other children are likely to remain interested longer.

MODIFYING STEREOTYPED BEHAVIORS
Although there are numerous studies concerning stereotyped behaviors in the blind, very

few are available on the deaf population. Murdoch (1996) surveyed 390 deaf and hearing impaired students in residential schools in England. He found that children who did not have additional disabilities did not display stereotypic behavior. In blind children this phenomenon is quite common. Troster *et al.* (1991a,b) showed that all 85 children in their study displayed at least one form of mannerism, and many had several. They reported that the range of behaviors expanded from the first to the second year of life and then decreased from age 3 up to enrollment in school. Eye poking and body rocking were found to be the most persistent. They discriminated between four settings in which the behaviors occurred: monotony, arousal, demand, and during feeding. They found that repetitive hand and finger movements, stereotypic manipulation of objects and making faces mainly took place in arousal situations, while eye poking, whimpering and sucking thumbs and fingers were mainly linked to monotony. This study is important because it implies that the type of behavior displayed can provide clues for effective intervention. When there is a great deal of eye poking it may be an indication that a change into a more active behavior pattern is required, while with excessive repetitive hand movements the level of stimulation may need to be reduced. In both instances the children appear to be withdrawing into themselves. When there is not enough to do they seek out something that is perceived as pleasant and mildly stimulating, and when there is too much going on that they cannot comprehend they revert to a simpler, predictable pattern. This can be acceptable if the behavior is not so prolonged that it takes the place of other, more functional behaviors, or if it is not socially inappropriate or harmful.

One of the reasons why deaf children are not reported to show stereotypic behavior may be because they have a better opportunity to observe what other children do and don't do. This does not mean that they do not have an urge towards certain repetitive behaviors, but the expression of those urges may be similar to the repetitive behavior patterns of the rest of the population and therefore they do not stand out. Many people who do not have a visual impairment find rocking back and forth soothing, hence the ample supply of rocking chairs. However, they do not generally sway back and forth in the middle of a room, because that would look odd. Children who cannot see what other children are doing tend to be less inhibited, because they have no visual models on which to judge their behavior, and they cannot see disapproving looks. 'Normalizing' some of the stereotypic behavior of blind children, such as finding a socially appropriate form for it, may be a more effective method of reducing a behavior that is perceived by other children as weird and that therefore could act as a social barrier. One should also be careful that functional behavior is not eliminated for appearances' sake. Some blind children put objects to their mouths for much longer than sighted children. This may be because the lips are very sensitive and can provide useful information about an object. Mouthing seems to be an important source of information for young blind children and should not necessarily be discouraged because it looks immature. Instead it could be used as a starting point for expanding the exploration and providing the child with more tactile, auditory and olfactory information. Only behavior patterns that no longer serve a purpose should be considered for elimination. Others, which are still functional but seem disruptive to others or inhibit social contacts, should be considered for adaptation rather than elimination, and often lend themselves well to a behavior modification program.

Although stereotypic behavior in deaf or hearing impaired children is not frequently described in the literature, there is a fair amount of information with regard to behavior problems and psychiatric disorders in this group. Prior *et al.* (1988) examined temperament and behavioral adjustment in 26 hearing impaired preschool children. They found that these children were rated by their mothers as having a more difficult temperament, but not a greater amount of behavior problems, than a normative group, while their teachers found them to be less well adjusted and more anxious. The mothers showed higher levels of anxiety and depression. Van Eldik (1994) found a greater incidence in internalizing and externalizing behavior problems in deaf boys as well as a greater incidence of problems overall, but reported that they were not more disturbed than hearing children. Vostanis *et al.* (1997) found a high rate of social maladjustment among deaf children who attended schools for the deaf. Hindley *et al.* (1994) also found that the rate of psychiatric disorder was higher in their study population of deaf and hearing impaired children than in a comparable group of hearing children. Rates of disorder were higher in the children who attended Hearing Impaired Units than in schools for the deaf. The Hearing Impaired Units were frequently attached to regular schools, and many of the children were teased and bullied, with their deafness as a focus. In the specialist schools, teasing and bullying also took place, but it was not centered around the impairment. Hindley *et al.* (1993) also cautioned against using an interviewer who is not fluent in sign language in psychiatric assessments of signing children and adolescents. Such a practice can mask the degree of the child's emotional problems. The need for mental health professionals who are able to sign is being recognized, and a separate discipline of psychology for the deaf has been proposed (Pollard 1996).

A higher incidence of psychiatric disorder has also been reported in visually impaired children (Jan *et al.* 1977). Autism especially has received a lot of attention (Preisler 1993, Hobson *et al.* 1997, Recchia 1997). This is not surprising, because congenitally blind young children often show a large number of the behavior characteristics associated with Autistic Disorder (DSM-IV: American Psychiatric Association 1994), such as stereotyped patterns of behavior, and qualitative impairments in communication and interaction. However, these characteristics may not have the same origin as in truly autistic children. The latter have access to the same sensory information as normally sighted children do. Blind children do not have the same information, and therefore some of the interactive patterns cannot be established in the same way. It may take them longer to establish a concept of the world that can be used effectively to interpret and share new information and experiences. Not only does the lack of vision make it more difficult for them to interpret all the information that accompanies social interactions, but also they may not be reinforced in their attempts at communication because their patterns of initiation are not familiar to the sighted person. The greatest risk for young severely sensory impaired children is that others give up trying to interact with them, because they seem to be so unresponsive. This could result in fewer opportunities for communication and exploration, which could delay the development of a symbolic understanding of the world around them, and this in turn could impair the ability to share abstract experiences. Deaf children, who do not have a problem with perception of the concrete world, may also have difficulty with the symbolic representation of their experiences, because they do not hear or see these experiences paired with the symbol frequently enough.

Self-reports, in the form of questionnaires or interviews, need to be treated with caution. Although the words may be understood, the concepts they represent may be interpreted differently.

CASE STUDY
Jonathan was described by his mother and his teachers as socially very isolated. He had no friends in school or in the neighborhood and interacted little with his older sister. Yet when he was asked how many close friends he had, he listed several. When questioned further, his best friend turned out to be the local postman. When he was asked how he would describe a best friend he responded, someone who comes to your house everyday.

Reports of abuse or maltreatment need to be treated equally cautiously, which does not mean that they are not to be taken seriously. It is very important that diagnoses or assessments of emotional and psychiatric disorders, social problems or learning disabilities are made by clinicians who have a thorough understanding of the developmental course of children with a sensory impairment. When this is not the case, sensory impaired children may run the risk of having problems which stem from the difference in access to the world around them labeled as a psychiatric condition or a learning disability. The resulting treatment may be totally ineffective, while if the root of the problem had been recognized, the environment and the interactive style of the people in it could have been modified to create a greater opportunity for exploration and sharing experiences. Conversely, care should also be taken that not all problems are automatically attributed to the sensory impairment. Deaf or blind children can also have additional mental health problems or learning disabilities that are not related to their sensory problems. They are just as likely to live in a dysfunctional family, perhaps more so, considering the greater amount of stress the disability may impose on families. Deafness or blindness in itself is not a source of grief or anger to the children with a congenital sensory impairment, because they do not have a clear concept of what it means to be otherwise. However, the social isolation that can result from such an impairment can cause distress and may require intervention. The course of the intervention will be more effective if it concentrates on greater acculturation with the child's peer group rather than on helping the child come to terms with the impairment. For children with a suddenly acquired impairment this is different and they, as well as their families, will need help with the emotional as well as the practical adjustment to the new condition. However, depending on the children's age at the onset of the impairment, they are likely to have a world perspective that is similar to that of children without an impairment, especially initially.

Conclusion
Addressing the problems of visually and hearing impaired children under the heading of sensory impairment has its disadvantages. This approach runs the risk of comparing them to children without a sensory impairment and implying that where they differ from them is where they share problems with each other. This kind of perspective leads to the

identification of problem areas, but not to solutions. In order to integrate a child with a sensory impairment more fully into society, it is imperative that their experience of the world be better understood. Longitudinal studies which concentrate on the culture of the congenitally deaf or blind may help in forging a bridge with those without a sensory impairment. Since deaf and blind children live in a world where the majority have a different world view from them, it is important that they learn to move in that world but not at the expense of sacrificing their own integrity and uniqueness. In order to develop a sense of cultural identity they will also need to share experiences and thoughts with those who share their sensory perspective. Children with partial impairments may run into even greater difficulty with trying to establish an identity, because they do not clearly belong to either culture. More research that specifically addresses the social and cultural needs in this group is highly desirable.

REFERENCES

American Psychiatric Association (1994) *Diagnostic and Statistical Manual of Mental Disorders, 4th Edn (DSM-IV)*. Washington, DC: APA.

Balkany, T., Hodges, A.V., Goodman, K.W. (1996) 'Ethics of cochlear implantation in young children.' *Otolaryngology, Head and Neck Surgery*, **114**, 748–755.

Brand, H.J., Coetzer, M.A. (1994) 'Parental response to their child's hearing impairment.' *Psychological Reports*, **75**, 1363–1368.

Cass, H.D., Sonksen, P., McConachie, H.R. (1994) 'Developmental setback in severe visual impairment.' *Archives of Disease in Childhood*, **70**, 192–196.

Cohen, N.L. (1994) 'The ethics of cochlear implants in young children.' *American Journal of Otology*, **15**, 1–2.

Davidson, I.F., Simmons, J.N. (1992) 'Young blind children: towards assessment for rehabilitation.' *International Journal of Rehabilitation Research*, **15**, 219–226.

Durieux-Smith, A., Delicati, D., Philips, A., Fitzpatric, E., Brewster, L. (1995) 'CASLPA position paper on cochlear implants in children.' *Journal of Speech and Language Pathology and Audiology*, **19**, 147–153.

Fish, L. (1983) 'Integrated development and maturation of the hearing system.' *British Journal of Audiology*, **17**, 137–154.

Fogel, A. (1997) 'Seeing and being seen.' *In:* Lewis, V., Collis, G.M. (Eds.) *Blindness and Psychological Development in Young Children*. Leicester: BPS Books, pp. 86–98.

Franco, F., Fogel, A., Messinger, D.S., Frazier, C.A. (1996) 'Cultural differences in physical contact between Hispanic and Anglo mother–infant dyads living in the United States.' *Early Development and Parenting*, **5**, 119–127.

Freeman, R.D., Carbin, C.F., Boese, R.J. (1981) *Can't Your Child Hear?* Baltimore: University Press.

Gaines, R., Halpern-Felsher, B.L. (1995) 'Language preference and communication development of a hearing and deaf twin pair.' *American Annals of the Deaf*, **140**, 47–55.

Groenveld, M. (1990) 'The dilemma of assessing the visually impaired child.' *Developmental Medicine and Child Neurology*, **32**, 1105–1113.

Hack, M., Breslau, N., Aram, D., Weissman, B., Klein, N., Borawski-Clark, E. (1992) 'The effect of very low birth weight and social risk on neurocognitive abilities at school age.' *Journal of Developmental and Behavioral Pediatrics*, **13**, 412–420.

Hindley, P., Hill, P., Bond, D. (1993) 'Interviewing deaf children, the interviewer effect: a research note.' *Journal of Child Psychology and Psychiatry*, **34**, 1461–1467.

—— —— McGuigan, S., Kitson, N. (1994) 'Psychiatric disorder in deaf and hearing impaired children and young people: a prevalence study.' *Journal of Child Psychology and Psychiatry*, **35**, 917–934.

Hobson, R.P., Brown, R., Minter, M.E., Lee, A. (1997) 'Autism revisited: the case of congenital blindness.' *In:* Lewis, V., Collis, G.M. (Eds.) *Blindness and Psychological Development in Young Children*. Leicester: BPS Books, pp. 99–115.

Iverson, J.M., Goldin-Meadow, S. (1997) 'What's communication got to do with it? Gesture in children blind from birth.' *Developmental Psychology*, **33**, 453–467.

Jan, J.E., Groenveld, M. (1993) 'Visual behaviours and behavioural adaptation to visual loss in children.' *Journal of Visual Impairment and Blindness*, **87**, 101–105.
—— Freeman, R.D., Scott, E.P. (1977) *Visual Impairment in Children and Adolescents*. New York: Grune & Stratton.
Johnson, M. (1987) *The Body in the Mind*. Chicago:University of Chicago Press.
Kalil, R.E. (1987) 'Synapse formation in the developing brain.' *Scientific American*, **261**, 76–85.
Konstantareas, M.M., Lampropoulou, V. (1995) 'Stress in Greek mothers with deaf children. Effects of child characteristics, family resources and cognitive set.' *American Annals of the Deaf*, **140**, 264–270.
Landau, B. (1997) 'Language and experience in blind children: retrospective and prospective.' In: Lewis, V., Collis, G.M. (Eds.) *Blindness and Psychological Development in Young Children*. Leicester: BPS Books, pp. 9–28.
Lane, H. (1993) *The Mask of Benevolence*. New York: Vintage Books.
Locke, J.L. (1997) 'Degrees of developmental and linguistic freedom.' *In:* Lewis, V., Collis, G.M. (Eds.) *Blindness and Psychological Development in Young Children*. Leicester: BPS Books, pp. 29–37.
McConachie, H. (1990) 'Early language development and severe visual impairment.' *Child: Care, Health and Development*, **16**, 55–61.
Meadow-Orlans, K.P., Smith-Gray, S., Dyssegaard, B. (1995) 'Infants who are deaf, or hard of hearing, with and without physical/cognitive disabilities.' *American Annals of the Deaf*, **140**, 279–286.
Miyamoto, R.T., Svirsky, M.A., Robbins, A.M. (1997) 'Enhancement of expressive language in prelingually deaf children with cochlear implants.' *Acta Otolaryngolica*, **117**, 154–157.
Murdoch, H. (1996) 'Stereotyped behaviors in deaf and hard of hearing children.' *American Annals for the Deaf*, **141**, 379–386.
Netelenbos, J.B., Savelsbergh, G.H. (1991) 'Localization of visual targets inside and outside the field of view: the effect of hearing loss.' *Journal of Child Psychology and Psychiatry*, **32**, 489–500.
Parving, A. (1984) 'Early detection and identification of congenital/early acquired hearing disability. Who takes the initiative?' *International Journal of Otorhinolaryngology*, **7**, 107–117.
Perez-Pereira, M. (1994) 'Imitations, repetitions, routines and the child's analysis of language: insights from the blind.' *Journal of Child Language*, **21**, 317–337.
Pollard, R.Q. (1996) 'Professional psychology and deaf people. The emergence of a discipline.' *American Psychologist*, **51**, 389–396.
Ponton, C.W., Don, M., Eggermont, J.J., Waring, M.D., Kwong, D., Masuda, A. (1996) 'Auditory system plasticity in children after long periods of complete deafness.' *Neuroreport*, **20**, 61–65.
Preisler, G.M. (1993) 'A descriptive study of blind children in nurseries with sighted children.' *Child: Care, Health and Development*, **19**, 295–315.
—— (1995) 'The development of communication in blind and in deaf infants—similarities and differences.' *Child: Care, Health and Development*, **21**, 79–110.
—— (1997) 'Social and emotional development of blind children: a longitudinal study.' *In:* Lewis, V., Collis, G.M. (Eds.) *Blindness and Psychological Development in Young Children*. Leicester: BPS Books, pp. 69–85.
Prendergast, S.G., McCollum, J.A. (1996) 'Let's talk: the effect of maternal hearing status on interactions with toddlers who are deaf.' *American Annals of the Deaf*, **141**, 11–18.
Prior, M.R., Glazner, J., Sanson, A., Debelle, G. (1988) 'Temperament and behavioural adjustment in hearing impaired children.' *Journal of Child Psychology and Psychiatry*, **29**, 209–216.
Recchia, S.L. (1997) 'Establishing intersubjective experience: developmental challenges for young children with congenital blindness and autism and their caregivers.' *In:* Lewis, V., Collis, G.M. (Eds.) *Blindness and Psychological Development in Young Children*. Leicester: BPS Books, pp. 116–129.
Robinson, G.C., Jan, J.E., Kinnis, C. (1987) 'Congenital blindness in children 1945–1984.' *American Journal of Diseases of Children*, **141**, 1321–1324.
Rose, D.E., Vernon, M., Pool, A.F. (1996) 'Cochlear implants in prelingually deaf children.' *American Annals of the Deaf*, **141**, 258–262.
Saigal, S., Szatmari, P., Rosenbaum, P., Campbell, D., King, S. (1990) 'Intellectual and functional status at school entry of children who weighed 1000 grams or less at birth: a regional perspective of births in the 1980s.' *Journal of Pediatrics*, **3**, 409–416.
Salvia, J., Ysseldyke, J.E. (1981) *Assessment in Special and Remedial Education*. Boston: Houghton Mifflin.
Schilling, L.S., DeJesus, E. (1993) 'Developmental issues in deaf children.' *Journal of Pediatric Health Care*, **7**, 161–166.

134

Shaw, J., Jamieson, J. (1997) 'Patterns of classroom discourse in an integrated, interpreted elementary school setting.' *American Annals for the Deaf*, **142**, 40–47.

Sloman, L., Springer, S., Vachon, M.L. (1993) 'Disordered communication and grieving in deaf member families.' *Family Process*, **32**, 171–183.

Stern, J.M. (1997) 'Offspring-induced nurturance: animal–human parallels.' *Developmental Psychobiology*, **31**, 19–37.

Swanson, L. (1997) 'Cochlear implants: the head-on collision between medical technology and the right to be deaf.' *Canadian Medical Association Journal*, **157**, 929–932

Troster, H., Bambring, M., Beelman, A. (1991a) 'Prevalence and situational causes of stereotyped behaviors in blind infants and preschoolers.' *Journal of Abnormal Child Psychology*, **19**, 569–590.

—— —— —— (1991b) 'The age dependence of stereotyped behavior in blind infants and preschoolers.' *Child: Care, Health and Development*, **17**, 137–157.

Tyler, R.S., Fryauf-Bertschy, H., Kelsay, D.M., Gantz, B.J., Woodworth, G.P. (1997) 'Speech perception by prelingually deaf children using cochlear implants.' *Otolaryngology, Head and Neck Surgery*, **117**, 180–187.

Van Eldik, T.T. (1994) 'Behavior problems with deaf Dutch boys.' *American Annals for the Deaf*, **139**, 394–399.

Vostanis, P., Hayes, M., Du Feu, M., Warren, J. (1997) 'Detection of behavioural and emotional problems in deaf children and adolescents: comparison of two scales.' *Child: Care Health and Development*, **23**, 233–246.

Youngson-Reilly, S., Tobin, M.J., Fielder, A.R. (1994) 'Patterns of professional involvement with parents of visually impaired children.' *Developmental Medicine and Child Neurology*, **36**, 449–458.

7
CEREBRAL PALSY

James Harris

'Cerebral palsy' (CP) is the accepted term for a group of nonprogressive disorders of motor control and posture that have behavioral, psychological and social implications for those affected, their families, and service providers. The cerebral palsies are made up of non-progressive motor disorders resulting from damage to the immature brain during pregnancy, at delivery, or in the early preschool years. They include a variety of neurologic conditions that have in common a developmental motor disorder (poor coordination, poor balance and abnormal movement patterns). The motor disorder may vary in cause, manifestations, severity of presentation, outcome and co-occurring conditions. Hence, the term 'cerebral palsy' is a general description and does not specify the type or severity of the motor deficit.

In addition to primary motor disorders, affected children may also have sensory, cognitive and behavioral disabilities. Approaches to dealing with such problems are discussed elsewhere in this book. The emphasis of the present chapter is on interventions, both family-based and behavioral. In order to understand how interventions may be used, one must under-stand the disorder, so detailed information is first provided on the causes and classification of CP.

In his classic study on 200 cases, William John Little (1861) distinguished CP from other causes of motor disability, attributing spastic rigidity to obstetric complications associated with lack of oxygen at the time of birth (see Accardo 1989). Because of his study, the disorder was subsequently referred to as 'Little's disease' (Accardo 1989). The current term cerebral 'palsy' (a contraction of the word 'paralysis'), was introduced by Sir William Osler in his 1889 book, *The Cerebral Palsies of Children*. An early clinical classification that has provided the basis for the later classifications was presented in 1897 by Sigmund Freud (a child and adult neurologist before turning to psychoanalysis) in his *Infantile Cerebral Paralysis* (see Accardo 1982). Freud emphasized prenatal influences and proposed that CP might be linked to intrauterine development of the fetus. Later, Crothers and Paine (1959), in *The Natural History of Cerebral Palsy*, refined the classification. The current system of classification of the clinical motor disorders was adopted by the American Academy of Cerebral Palsy in the 1950s (Minear 1956). Early interventions focused on the prevention and early treatment of CP, utilizing physical therapy. Current treatments address neurobehavioral interventions for the movement disorder, behavior management of the child, and family adaptation.

CP becomes evident during the developmental period when brain growth is most rapid. Although nonprogressive, it is not an unchanging disorder. Thus, changes in the movement disorder occur as the brain continues to grow (Mutch *et al.* 1992). A floppy (hypotonic) infant may develop spastic or rigid CP by the preschool years. Depending on the extent of brain involvement, CP may be mild, moderate or severe. In some cases, there is a gradual improvement in the movement disorder, but other cases show limited progress and reach a plateau. Many of those afflicted require bracing and surgery.

How common is CP?

It is estimated that moderate-to-severe CP occurs in one out of every 1000 births and that milder CP occurs in up to five in 1000 births (Stanley and Alberman 1984). The incidence has remained constant over the past 30 years despite the fact that management of pregnancy, delivery and care of the newborn has improved (Stanley 1987). This is because medical advances have led to the survival of low birthweight infants who previously would have died, and many of these surviving low birthweight infants have developed CP. Extremely low birthweight infants are also at greater risk for mental retardation and learning disabilities.

Spastic CP, characterized by rigidity in muscles leading to stiffness and restricted movements, is the most frequent type and accounts for approximately 80 per cent of cases, followed by athetosis (tremors, unsteadiness, and poor coordination) in 10 per cent, while the remaining children have mixed forms (Grether *et al.* 1992, Hack *et al.* 1994, Miller *et al.* 1995).

Because of the instability of the diagnosis when first detected in infancy, the age at which CP should be diagnosed is debated. Some have suggested that brain damage occurring before the age of 3 years should be used as a guideline, but others propose the age of 5. By using a later age of onset, children with acquired CP occurring from infection or trauma may also be included. Despite the severity of the condition, the survival rate has remained high for individuals who complete the neonatal period, reaching 88 per cent in the 1940s and '50s (Cohen and Mustacchi 1966).

What are the causes?

The National Collaborative Perinatal Project (Nelson and Ellenberg 1986, Nelson 1988) concluded that the majority of CP cases did not have specifically defined causes. Thus, prenatal, perinatal and genetic factors must all be considered in determining the cause. Because multiple brain regions are involved in the coordination of muscle activity, several sites may be involved. Although brain hemorrhage associated with preterm birth (Powell *et al.* 1988a,b; Kuban and Leviton 1994) may be the most common cause, inflammatory disease of the brain and its membrane covering, stroke, head injury or poisoning also may be causal factors. However, no known cause, unrecognized events during pregnancy, or unknown genetic abnormality is recorded in 20–30 per cent of cases. In the first year of life, central nervous system infections have been reported to account for 6 per cent of cases (Naeye *et al.* 1989), while about 2 per cent have been attributed to genetic factors (Hughes and Newton 1992).

Abnormal migration of neurons in the brain, occurring between 7 and 16 weeks of gestation, could lead to motor dysfunction, seizures, and learning and behavioral problems. Both environmental and genetic factors at sensitive developmental periods may affect neuronal migration.

137

How is it classified?

CP is generally classified according to the type of movement disorder (spastic, athetoid or hypotonic) or by the areas of the body that are involved (legs only, one arm and one leg, or both arms and both legs). Movement problems are divided into two main groups, the spastic types and the nonspastic types. Classification by limb involvement is applied only to the spastic types. Associated conditions, such as learning disability, are described in a supplemental classification (Minear 1956, Bax 1964). Because all forms of CP have a hypotonic phase, the initial classification of a case must be tentative until a syndrome has emerged. The classification may be difficult because of subtle abnormalities and mixed features.

NONSPASTIC (EXTRAPYRAMIDAL) TYPES

The nonspastic types of CP are subdivided into choreoathetoid, dystonic, ataxic and rigid forms. There is considerable variability in expression, so that the movement disorder may vary with activity level, with emotional arousal, and when muscle tension to carry out an activity is required. During sleep or relaxation, symptoms are generally less intense.

Athetosis refers to a lack of muscle control with involuntary movements involving various muscle groups. Affected individuals may appear contorted, stiff, or at other times in continuous motion. Speech also may be dysarthric, *i.e.* difficulty is experienced in co-ordinating and articulating words. Chorea refers to involuntary jerking movements involving the face, tongue and limbs, especially the extremities, and, in some individuals, the trunk. These movements are rapid, irregular, and become more pronounced during voluntary movement. Choreoathetoid is the term used when chorea and athetosis occur together.

Dystonia is a type of movement disorder that involves prolonged muscle contractions causing twisting and repetitive movements or abnormal postures. The dystonic form of CP generally involves extreme involuntary movements where the body and/or the arms and legs are forced into fixed postures by strong muscle contraction.

Ataxic (balance and coordination problems), rigid and atonic types of CP are much less common. Ataxic CP involves the cerebellum; thus, problems with muscle tone are the primary features. Hypotonia and severe motor delays are present in childhood, but with time, functioning may improve. Poor muscle tone is characteristic, and there may be associated bone deformities. Besides these, there are mixed types of the nonspastic forms.

Individuals with nonspastic forms of CP are thought to have damage to the basal ganglia of the brain. The cerebrum is usually not involved, so learning disability is less common than in the spastic types. Both spastic and nonspastic forms may be diagnosed in the same person.

SPASTIC (PYRAMIDAL) TYPES

Spasticity is characterized by the inability of a muscle to relax, with increased muscle tone and persistent muscle contraction in the involved muscle groups. The neurologic findings vary little with attempted movement, with emotion or during sleep and are associated with abnormal reflexes. Subtypes of spasticity are classified according to the number of limbs involved: monoplegia (one limb), diplegia (two limbs), triplegia (three limbs), quadriplegia (all four limbs), and hemiplegia (an arm and a leg on the same side of the body). As children with spastic CP grow older, increased muscle tone may lead to contractures and associated musculoskeletal deformities that may require orthopedic surgery. Moreover, abnormal reflexes, such as primitive reflexes (the persistence of brainstem-mediated movement patterns that are present at birth and normally disappear between 3 and 6 months of age), may lead to persistent problems in posture and movement. There may be variability in upper and lower limb involvement. In hemiplegia, the upper limbs are frequently more impaired than the lower ones. In diplegia, all four limbs can be involved, although the upper limbs may show only minimal involvement. In quadriplegia, the upper limbs may be less impaired than the lower ones; however, there is still severe involvement of all limbs. Monoplegia and triplegia are less commonly diagnosed and may be variations of hemiplegia and quadriplegia.

A great deal has to be learned about the natural history of CP, particularly in regard to how the severity of the condition in early life relates to subsequent outcome. To do so, in addition to the methods of classification described above, it is necessary to take into account ambulatory status, impairments in voluntary control of movement, muscle tone and reflex patterns. Palisano *et al.* (1997) have proposed a classification based on current adaptive functioning. In doing so, they have used the International Classification of Impairments, Disabilities and Handicaps (WHO 1980), which takes account of the severity of the disorder and of abilities and limitations in gross motor function. Their classification system can be used by professionals and families to determine a child's needs for management, to monitor progress and to compare the results of various interventions, as well as to develop databases. The authors anticipate that such a system may be used to help parents and professionals predict later motor function. A classification based on adaptive functioning may also be used to establish realistic goals for behavior programs.

The system includes a five-level classification system of motor function. This is based on self-initiated movement, with particular emphasis on sitting (truncal control) and walking. The focus is to establish which of the five levels best represents the child's present abilities and limitations in motor function, with emphasis on her/his usual performance in school and in the community. Each level represents the highest level of mobility that a child may accomplish between 6 and 12 years of age. The classification emphasizes functioning abilities rather than limitations. The levels are as follows:

Level I: walks without restrictions; limitations in more advanced gross motor skills.

Level II: walks without assistive devices; limitations in walking outdoors and in the community.

Level III: walks with assistive mobility devices; limitations in walking outdoors and in the community.

Level IV: self-mobility with limitations; children are transported or use power mobility outdoors and in the community.

Level V: self-mobility is severely limited, even with the use of assistive technology.

How does CP change over time?
For children who experience lesions or abnormalities of the brain arising in the early stages

of its development and have subsequent involvement of the motor system, sequential changes have been documented as the motor disorder evolves over time. For example, early infantile hypotonia (floppiness) may progress to spasticity in early childhood. Resistance to movement of the forearm, ankle and knee as a result of an abnormal stretch reflex is the earliest motor finding. For spastic diplegia, symptoms are first demonstrated in the legs; these may be manifested with leg extension or scissoring when the child is vertically suspended. The increased muscle tone is present when the child is placed down to walk. In spastic hemiplegia, symptoms are first demonstrated in the arms and expressed as unequal muscle tone. Difficulty with feeding may become apparent. The duration of hypotonia is variable, lasting 6–17 months or longer; the longer it lasts, the greater the severity of the disability. The term 'hypotonic CP' is used if it lasts longer than three years.

Hypotonia may be followed by dystonia. For example, when the infant extends her/his head, abnormal extensor neck postures that are rigid may become apparent. Such episodes present from 2 to 12 months of age. In nonspastic forms of CP, hypotonia is accompanied by immature (primitive) postural reflexes, such as the asymmetric tonic neck reflex (reflex arm extension when the head is turned), that persist longer than in those with spastic forms of CP. The earliest sign of dysfunction is finger posturing, which becomes apparent when the infant reaches for an object and may be evident by 9 months of age.

With increasing age, not only do the motor consequences of early birth injury become more evident, but so too do cognitive, academic and behavioral problems, as well as perceptual problems and hyperactivity. The degree of disability is wide—from mild spasticity, where ambulation is possible in an individual who may be cognitively impaired, to athetoid conditions with speech problems, where the individual may have average or above-average intelligence but be essentially nonverbal and dependent on the family for care, requiring special communication devices to interact with others.

Other disabling conditions associated with CP
The nonmotor disabling conditions associated with CP include mental retardation, sensory impairment of vision and hearing, language disorders, specific learning disorders and other cognitive impairments (Capute and Accardo 1991). These, together with psychological and psychiatric problems (social, emotional and family dysfunction) limit the extent to which rehabilitation is possible and will require psychosocial, psychological and behavioral interventions in their own right.

Cognitive difficulties are often the most seriously disabling problems for children with CP. These may be further complicated by speech and motor disability in the preschool years, and academic and learning difficulties once they begin school. Visual–perceptual problems and speech and hearing impairments will also influence learning. Recognition and appropriate intervention for associated disabilities is critical to prevent behavioral problems. Communication disorders are therefore particularly important to remediate; speech synthesizers and communication boards are required for nonverbal children to facilitate interpersonal communication. It is also essential to be aware that older children may face new and more stressful problems, such as the continuing need for surgery, bracing, and the use of other adaptive equipment.

Capute and Accardo (1991) describe disabling conditions that commonly accompany the various types of CP. Spastic hemiplegia is often associated with seizures, growth arrest, and sensory deficits involving specific brain regions (*e.g.* a visual field abnormality). Spastic diplegia may be associated with strabismus. Spastic quadriplegia is often associated with epilepsy, mental retardation and speech articulation problems, as well as strabismus. Choreo-athetoid forms are associated with mental retardation, auditory impairment and speech problems. Finally, quadriplegia tends to be associated with seizures, movement abnormalities, and cognitive impairment that is more severe than in hemiplegia or diplegia (Grether *et al.* 1992).

INTELLECTUAL DISABILITY (MENTAL RETARDATION)
Intellectual disability occurs in 30–60 per cent of people with CP and is among the most important factors influencing vulnerability to environmental stressors and psychiatric disorder (Evans *et al.* 1990, Rumeau-Rouquette *et al.* 1992). The degree of cognitive impairment varies widely and will obviously determine the level at which the child should be taught. However, multiple physical disabilities make testing very difficult, and a variety of tests may be needed. Blair and Stanley (1985), in their survey of 1000 6-year-olds, found an average IQ of 68 with a range broader than that of the general population. Children with ataxia (balance and coordination problems) showed the greatest variability; those with athetoid and spastic types showed less impairment, although those with spasticity were more cognitively impaired than the athetoid group. The intellectual deficit was greater in those with spastic quadriplegia than in those with paraplegia or spastic hemiparesis.

ACADEMIC DIFFICULTIES
Assessment of neuropsychological and academic skills is essential for the identification of strengths and weaknesses in learning. Reading disability is a consequence of deficits in language processing, visual perception, auditory processing and sequencing. An individualized education program is crucial to bring out the potential of each affected child and to prevent behavioral problems linked to repeated failure.

How is CP assessed?
An integrated approach to evaluation requires the intervention of an interdisciplinary team who will conduct pediatric, neurologic, psychiatric, orthopedic, ophthalmologic, dental, psychological, educational, physical therapy, occupational therapy, social work, and speech and language evaluations. Because cognitive ability may be difficult to assess due to the motor disability and the associated language disorder, standardized testing needs to be adapted to reflect the child's particular capacities and deficits.

Besides the standard neurologic examination, a neurodevelopmental examination is needed to evaluate motor development. Determining whether there is a permanent movement disorder can be difficult since early motor signs may diminish or resolve. There also may be a reticence to diagnose CP during the first six months of life, especially as motor delays may resolve with maturation in some infants between 6 and 18 months. Because of maturational changes, follow-up for motor disorders must continue into the school-age years (Hack 1994).

Noninvasive brain imaging techniques may be utilized to expand assessment methods. For example, ultrasound of the brain is used in the early diagnosis of preterm infants. Cranial ultrasound may be carried out through the open anterior fontanelle in preterm infants to identify lesions that may correlate with later motor disability. Computed tomography (CT) and magnetic resonance imaging (MRI) may be indicated to evaluate structural changes in the brain (Volpe 1992).

How is the parent–child relationship affected?
ATTUNEMENT/ATTACHMENT

Temperamental and physical features related to brain dysfunction may interfere with the establishment of parent–infant attunement and attachment and thus affect early social developmental milestones (Cox and Lambrenos 1992). Psychological attunement between child and parent is particularly affected by CP. This attunement, which involves the usual coordination of infant bodily movement with the mother's voice tone and gestures (interactional synchrony), may be impossible. Similarly, the infant's ability to move away from the parent to explore the environment and then return to a secure base is limited. This, along with parent–child communication problems, may affect attachment and the later development of 'working models' of relationships, as described below.

The persistence of primitive postural reflexes and abnormal cries also interferes with the establishment of an attachment relationship. Common problems for parents include misinterpretation of reflexes, such as the tonic neck reflex (reflex arm extension when the head is turned). This response can be particularly confusing to parents, and some mothers have interpreted it as an intentional effort to push them away. Affected children may also produce a high-pitched cry associated with spasmodic arching of the neck and back (opisthotonic movements) that can elicit considerable parental anxiety. Physical therapy can help to teach effective holding and handling techniques that allow the inhibition of these reflex activities so as to facilitate attachment and, to some extent, normalize the parent–child relationship.

WORKING MODELS OF RELATIONSHIPS

Normal child development in its earliest phases results in the internalization of cognitive 'working models' of the caregivers (Bowlby 1988). To facilitate the establishment of working models for children with CP, interpersonal communication is critical and communication devices are essential. Positive internal working models of parent–child relationships provide the security to cope with separation during the early school years. With maturation and increased awareness of their disability, a positive sense of self that has emerged from positive working models can help children to cope with stress and stigmatization.

Common behavior problems
McDermott et al. (1996) conducted a population-based analysis of behavior problems in children with CP. Behavior problems were reported to occur five times more often in children with CP (25.5 per cent) than in those with no known health problems (5.4 per cent), and were particularly common in children with CP and mental retardation. Specific problem

behaviors identified were overdependency, 'acting headstrong' and hyperactivity. It is important to note, however, that despite the increased frequency of such problems in children with CP, the majority did not have significant behavior problems. In another study of 98 children with CP, Breslau (1990) found that the main problems were social isolation and challenging behaviors such as oppositionality and dependency.

Research is needed to focus on protective factors related to the child's physical status and psychosocial environment that may reduce the risk for the development of these problems. Such factors might include social support networks for children and families, carefully selected school placements, and behavior programs to encourage independence. Further efforts are also needed to assess the effectiveness of parental anticipatory guidance (ongoing advice about what to expect in the future), the impact of physical, occupational, and speech and language interventions, and the outcome of psychological counseling and behavior therapy for children and families.

How does the family adapt to the child's disability?

Because parents are active participants in the child's care they must be confident about the diagnosis and fully informed about the treatment plan. As noted above, CP and its associated features vary from one individual to the next, and the extent of involvement will affect parents' adjustment to the disability. Early diagnosis by a sensitive clinician can be crucial to the adaptation process. Unfortunately, however, even though the parents may express concern about a floppy infant, the physician will often suggest that they wait several months or more to confirm the diagnosis. Such delays can be extremely stressful and the situation may be further complicated by the parents' misunderstandings about their child's behavior.

To ensure the best developmental outcome, it is essential to help the parents work through their distress and adjust to the child's disability. Comprehensive care is needed to aid in the adjustment process. In particular, ongoing advice and information about what to expect in the future regarding the associated brain damage, cognitive deficits and learning disabilities can help to reduce vulnerability to social and psychiatric problems.

Interviewing the parent

The family history includes queries about developmental disorders and behavioral and psychiatric disturbance in other family members. The most common psychological factors that affect the parents' adjustment to the child are denial of the disability, self-blame, blaming of others, guilt, depression and dependency, and these will all need to be dealt with (Richmond 1972, Mac Keith 1976). The interview begins by clarifying the extent of denial: do the parents have a realistic understanding of the nature and extent of the disability? Their denial of the seriousness of the disability may place the child at risk for inappropriate or inadequate treatment. The interviewer inquires about whom the parents talk to when they have concerns about their child: do they have a close confiding relationship with one another, or are they socially isolated? Next, questions are posed regarding guilt: whom do they feel is to blame for the child's condition? Assessment of self-blame and guilt is an important issue because it may herald an emerging depressive disorder. Parents often experience self-blame regarding their child-rearing skills and, in some instances, shame for having a disabled child. A final area to be covered in the interview is the parents' sense of adequacy as parents. Do they feel secure in their ability to care for their child, or have they become increasingly dependent on others? Do they anxiously, automatically and unquestioningly follow advice from others? Do they regard themselves as helpless? When this is the case, overwhelmed parents commonly make frequent telephone calls about minor illnesses and may make requests for the physician to make decisions unrelated to treatment of CP. It is not only their own caregiving skills but also those of others that concern parents. Do they feel that team members can be trusted to complete procedures that they do themselves at home? Parents may criticize team members as a consequence of their anxiety, and will benefit from being given the opportunity to ventilate their feelings directly.

After determining the degree of the parents' acceptance of the disability, the parents' future plans for the affected child as well as for their other children must be considered. It is particularly important to establish if there is a genetic basis for the condition and whether there are implications for future family planning. With successful adaptation, parents can be helped to regain the capacity to invest energy in caring for each other and other family members and to make appropriate future plans for their affected child.

Interviewing the disabled child
The interview with the child requires that both the child's developmental level and her/his means of most effective communication be considered. Patience and adequate time are needed to understand the child's speech. A letter board, speech synthesizer or individualized communication procedure may be necessary for an effective interview. Assistance from a speech pathologist may be required initially until familiarity with the communication equipment develops. With the use of a communication device, the interview proceeds as it would with another child of equivalent mental age.

Common problems in the child's adaptation
When appropriate physical and psychological supports are provided, the child with CP may have an active school and family life. However, adjustment problems are common and must be considered in management. Hurley and Sovner (1987) found that dependency and passivity, hopelessness and frustration, lack of social competence, and guilt and shame were the most common concerns.

Due to the motor disability, the child with CP may become excessively dependent on others and demonstrate a lack of assertiveness. Such dependency is often the result of others providing for her/his physical needs over a long period of time. With constant care the child may lack the initiative to develop self-help skills. This attitude of dependency can be fostered by the parents who find it difficult to adapt to the child's disability. Excessive parental guilt may result in overprotection and an unwillingness to allow age-appropriate independence. Appropriate psychological support is needed to assist parents in fostering this independence.

Particularly for the higher-functioning individual with athetoid CP, the inability to carry out tasks easily and with fluidity of movement can lead to considerable frustration. Moreover, the sense of being different from others becomes more apparent with age. Being a victim of an incurable condition requires a focus on tasks that the child can master.

Physical problems that are difficult to control, such as dribbling food or drooling saliva, urinary incontinence, and the movement disorder itself commonly result in social isolation. In addition, social competence is often confounded by social–emotional learning disability, *i.e.* problems focusing attention on and understanding interpersonal social cues. School failure may be the consequence of learning disabilities that lead to difficulties in completing school work.

Social stigma is an ongoing challenge that is linked to physical appearance, difficulty completing activities of daily living, and lack of attention to social cues. Further stigma arises when higher-functioning children with athetoid CP are misdiagnosed as being mentally retarded. Social rejection is a particularly sensitive issue following the onset of adolescence, when peer group relationships become more important. In adulthood, stigma, social rejection and discrimination may occur in the work place.

Like parents, children may experience a sense of guilt and shame regarding their disability. As they mature, they are likely to become increasingly aware of the burdens of the disability as it relates to both physical care and cost. A positive parental attitude toward the disability is therefore essential to help the child work through these feelings. As the adolescent moves into adulthood, the need for services in the community increases, and at this stage, greater social support is required for both child and parents.

What psychiatric disorders should be considered?

Psychiatric disorders in individuals with CP include those associated with physical disability, such as adjustment disorder, personality trait disturbance, difficult temperament, and major psychiatric diagnoses.

Brain damage is a major vulnerability factor in the establishment of psychiatric and severe behavioral disorders (Rutter *et al.* 1970). However, the mechanisms linking brain dysfunction to behavioral abnormality remain uncertain. Breslau (1990) questioned the mechanism of how brain dysfunction leads to behavioral disturbance—is it direct or does brain dysfunction increase the child's vulnerability to environmental stressors?

Persons with CP have increased rates of mood changes, irritability, attention deficits, impulsiveness, and limited skills in social problem-solving. Breslau (1990) interviewed 157 children with CP or multiple disabilities and 339 randomly selected controls, along with their parents. Depressive symptoms and inattention were significantly associated with the physical disabilities. Family environment was an important variable for depression in both groups, but inattention was not, and difficult temperament was demonstrated to be an important vulnerability factor. Breslau reported that parental/child problems, alone or with a difficult temperament, were also associated with psychiatric disorder.

Parental overprotection is a risk factor for separation anxiety disorder. Inadequate limit-setting increases the risk of developing oppositional behavior disorder. Brief psychotic reactions may occur in response to stress and must be distinguished from schizophrenia. Major mental illnesses, such as mood disorder and schizophrenia, may appear in adolescence or in early adult life in people with CP just as they do in the general population. Mood disorder is of concern, because major depression may go unrecognized or be misdiagnosed as an adjustment disorder when the involved person has difficulty participating in a psychiatric interview. Moreover, individuals with mood disorder are at greater risk for accidents, such as falls.

What constitutes a comprehensive management program?

Comprehensive treatment includes general pediatric supervision, psychoeducational assessment, appropriate school programs (Kohn 1990), orthopedic management (Bleck 1987), physical and occupational therapy, psychological support and behavior therapy. Advances in rehabilitation technology include the use of orthotics (braces), robotics, mobility and seating devices, and up-to-date computer interfaces for the control of devices. Assistive and augmentative communication devices are critical for many aspects of the child's development (*e.g.* being able to make choices and understanding cause–effect relationships) and should be introduced as early as possible. Levitt (1995) provides an extensive description of the treatment of the motor disorder in CP. McCormick *et al.* (1993) discuss early educational interventions in low birthweight infants. A comprehensive approach to parent education also includes well-written educational materials (Blasco *et al.* 1983, Miller *et al.* 1995).

A comprehensive approach provides education in carrying out the routine tasks of toileting, feeding, dressing and transferring the child from one place to another. Feeding can be a particular problem for the parent of a child with CP, and help is needed in behavior management to avoid prolonged feeding sessions. Tongue thrust, *i.e.* forceful tongue protrusion on stimulation, may interfere with breast and bottle feeding. Moreover, reflexive biting may take place when the gums are stimulated. To help overcome such problems, techniques that help to position the infant to optimize muscle tone by inhibiting excessive tone or muscle extensions, and methods for introducing the nipple or teat and supporting the jaw can all be taught to parents.

Incontinence is another major management problem. Psychological, cognitive, neurologic and neuromuscular factors must be considered. Because toileting is difficult and the child or adolescent may be reluctant to cooperate, behaviorally based interventions may be needed. In some instances, incontinence occurs sporadically and may be related to spasticity of the bladder. An intermittently incontinent patient is sometimes interpreted as showing a lack of motivation rather than having a physical disorder. Such children may, in turn, characterize themselves as lazy or feel hopeless about their lack of control and will require understanding and support of their dilemma.

BEHAVIORAL INTERVENTIONS

Behavioral approaches for children with CP, as for any other child, can range from procedures that focus only on overt behavior to cognitive behavioral approaches that emphasize learning better self-control. Behavioral approaches in CP are helpful for movement disorders (Horn *et al.* 1995), feeding problems, toileting problems, enhancing social skills, improving activities of daily living, academic task mastery, and dealing with challenging behaviors (particularly aggression and self-injurious behavior). Behavioral approaches can also improve motivation to complete tasks appropriate to their developmental level (Carr 1982). Behavioral strategies may be used to reduce dependency, to reduce rates of aggression and oppositional behavior, and to provide appropriate consequences for 'headstrong' children.

As for any other condition, an applied behavior analysis is necessary to clarify environmental influences on behavior and the conditions under which the problems occur, and to assess their frequency, duration and intensity. Family members are interviewed and asked to specify their goals for treatment and their willingness to participate in intervention. The therapist can help them to identify antecedents and consequences for the target behaviors and to review the effectiveness of management techniques that may have been used in the past.

As noted elsewhere in this book, behavior therapy programs utilize both behavior enhancement and behavior reduction strategies. Behavior enhancement procedures are preferred because they help to reduce undesirable behaviors by promoting adaptive approaches to overcome problems. Behavior enhancement is established by increasing the probability that socially appropriate and adaptive behaviors will occur. Moreover, as adaptive behaviors increase and the child receives greater reinforcement, further undesirable behaviors are likely to reduce in frequency. One example of behavioral enhancement is the use of differential reinforcement procedures. For instance, the caregiver might show approval for sharing but ignore or withdraw social approval when the child refuses to share. Types of differential reinforcement, all involving positive reinforcement, include differential reinforcement of appropriate or alternative behavior (DRA), differential reinforcement of incompatible behavior (DRI), and differential reinforcement of other behaviors (DRO). In contrast, behavior reduction procedures reduce maladaptive behaviors by establishing undesirable consequences for them when they occur. An example is the 'time-out' procedure which involves the removal of access to positive reinforcement, *e.g.* in time-out the child is not permitted to participate in a preferred activity. Time-outs must be consistently applied and of brief duration; lengthy time-outs may lose their effectiveness. Another behavior reduction procedure is referred to as 'response cost'. This involves the loss of a positive reinforcer, such as loss of a privilege, or the introduction of a penalty. However, the use of relatively mild punishment techniques of this kind with children who already have to cope with so many difficulties in their lives poses considerable ethical issues. Of course, at times they may be necessary, especially when behaviors are particularly disruptive or limit the child's ability to make progress in other areas. Whenever possible, though, positive reinforcement is preferable, and the techniques described in detail in Chapter 4 may also be used very successfully in children with CP.

In developing a behavioral intervention, a sensitive orientation to the affected person should be maintained to foster social attachment. McGee (1988) has identified three problematic attitudes of a therapist or parent (the overprotective, the authoritarian, and the mechanistic) that may interfere with effective behavior management. An overprotective attitude may be benevolent but makes few demands on the child and may thereby restrict the development of independence by limiting community experiences. An authoritarian approach may result in behavior reduction or suppression without establishing the necessary personal relationship that provides motivation for sustained compliance. An impersonal mechanistic attitude may highlight conformity to routines without allowing a meaningful interpersonal bond to be established. McGee suggests that the most appropriate attitude is one that focuses on interpersonal engagement with the child, with the goal of establishing an attachment bond.

The therapist is warm, nonjudgmental and socially interactive. Such an approach is more likely to engender a sense of security, consistency and positive expectations of success in the child. The therapist engages the child, and inappropriate behavior is ignored, interrupted and redirected, while positive behaviors are reinforced.

When behavioral approaches are used in motor habilitation, outcomes must be carefully evaluated. Harris (1993) supports the use of single-subject designs to evaluate outcome. An example of a specific program is presented by Horn *et al.* (1995). These authors carried out an experimental analysis of a neurobehavioral intervention. Using multiple baseline interventions in four children with CP (ages 21–34 months), they found that targeted experience can influence motor development, stressing the importance of behavioral intervention for children with motor disorder. They also found that functional activity and repetition can facilitate the acquisition and expression of underlying motor components, *e.g.* increased flexion control. They suggest that a focus on acquisition and expression of motor components may be a better means of assessing the outcome of intervention, rather than focusing on the full acquisition of a motor milestone. They point out that practice can enhance the development of basic neuromotor patterns, in contrast to the findings of Palmer *et al.* (1988) which suggest no discernible effects of physical therapy on the motor development of children with CP. Horn *et al.* emphasize that, in most intervention studies they reviewed, generalization to community settings was not provided or was not adequately measured. They suggest that neurobehavioral intervention is a primary intervention to develop early motor skills and deserves further experimental research.

OTHER PSYCHOLOGICAL TREATMENTS

Psychotherapy must be individually tailored and targeted to the associated features of the disorder. Communication devices, *e.g.* communication boards and other special devices to improve communication, are essential. Even then, patience is required for effective therapeutic interventions, and help from family members must often be elicited in interpreting the disabled person's speech.

Psychotherapy initially focuses on establishing children's understanding of the current problem and of the nature of their disability, and their feelings about how it affects their lives. Subsequently, better self-control and self-regulation and learning to accept responsibility for their own behavior are addressed. To do so, problem-solving techniques are utilized to help the child understand consequences, recognize emotional states, acknowledge differences in another person's point of view from one's own, and appreciate the effect of one's behavior on others.

Therapeutic approaches to parents include crisis intervention techniques, anticipatory guidance and preventive interventions. Anticipatory guidance is needed at times of predictable crisis, including the time of initial diagnosis, entering school, becoming an adolescent, and leaving home after completion of schooling. Preventive interventions are required when crises occur. One common crisis is the recognition at school entry that the child has additional cognitive disabilities. When preventive interventions are unsuccessful, short-term psychotherapy for the parents may be needed. Such psychotherapy emphasizes adaptation to the current crisis and working through denial, guilt, projection and dependency.

Drug Treatment

Finally, drug treatment may be required for the patient, either as a short-term intervention or a longer-term treatment depending on the presenting diagnosis. The parent and the child should be actively involved in treatment whenever medication is suggested for the child. A careful baseline neurologic examination is required before initiating treatment, and the patient's level of understanding of the effects of medication must be taken into account in monitoring drug side-effects.

Summary

CP and associated disabling conditions, particularly mental retardation, continue to be important disorders requiring early intervention, especially given the increased survival of affected infants.

Comprehensive treatment for both infants and children requires familiarity with the different types of CP, knowledge of the cognitive and other associated disabilities, and recognition of the child's and family's adaptation to the disability. With maturation, changes in function and in the degree of motor impairment occur and associated disabilities may become more apparent. Parental anticipatory guidance is needed at times of predictable family crisis such as the time of initial diagnosis, the preschool years, school entry, adjustment at adolescence, and at the time of leaving home. Parents may need help to appreciate the physical basis of difficulties with feeding, continence or mobility. They may also need support to avoid becoming overly protective and to help increase the child's independence. For children and adolescents with CP, behavioral approaches may be used to overcome a wide range of difficulties including feeding and toileting problems, and to enhance neuromotor training, academic task mastery, and social and daily living skills.

REFERENCES

Accardo, P.J. (1982) 'Freud on diplegia: commentary and translation.' *American Journal of Diseases of Children*, **136**, 452–456.
—— (1989) 'William John Little (1810–1894) and cerebral palsy in the nineteenth century.' *Journal of the History of Medicine and Allied Sciences*, **44**, 56–71.
Bax, M.C.O. (1964) 'Terminology and classification of cerebral palsy.' *Developmental Medicine and Child Neurology*, **6**, 295–297.
Blair, E., Stanley, F. (1985) 'Interobserver agreement in the classification of cerebral palsy.' *Developmental Medicine and Child Neurology*, **27**, 615–622.
Blasco, P., Baumgartner, M., Mathes, B. (1983) 'Literature for parents of children with cerebral palsy.' *Developmental Medicine and Child Neurology*, **25**, 642–647.
Bleck, E.E. (1987) *Orthopedic Management in Cerebral Palsy. Clinics in Developmental Medicine No. 99/100.* London: Mac Keith Press.
Bowlby, J. (1988) 'Developmental psychiatry comes of age.' *American Journal of Psychiatry*, **145**, 1–10.
Breslau, N. (1990) 'Does brain dysfunction increase children's vulnerability to environmental stress?' *Archives of General Psychiatry*, **47**, 15–20.
Capute, A.J., Accardo, P.J. (1991) *Developmental Disabilities in Infancy and Childhood.* Baltimore, MD: Brookes.
Carr, J. (1982) 'A behavioural approach to problems of motivation in the spina bifida child.' *Zeitschrift für Kinderchirurgie*, **37**, 184–186.
Cohen, P., Mustacchi, P. (1966) 'Survival in cerebral palsy.' *Journal of the American Medical Association*, **195**, 462. *(Editorial.)*

Cox, A.O., Lambrenos, K. (1992) 'Childhood physical disability and attachment.' *Developmental Medicine and Child Neurology*, **34**, 1037–1046.

Crothers, B., Paine, R.S. (1959) *The Natural History of Cerebral Palsy*. (Reprinted 1990 as *Classics in Developmental Medicine No. 2*. London: Mac Keith Press.)

Evans, P.M., Evans, S.J.W., Alberman, E. (1990) 'Cerebral palsy: why we must plan for survival.' *Archives of Disease in Childhood*, **65**, 1329–1333.

Freud, S. (1897) *Infantile Cerebral Paralysis*. (*Reprinted* 1968 by University of Miami Press, Coral Gables, FL.)

Grether, J.K., Cummins, S.K., Nelson, K.B. (1992) 'The California Cerebral Palsy Project.' *Pediatric and Perinatal Epidemiology*, **6**, 339–351.

Hack, M., Taylor, H.G., Klein, N., Eiben, R., Schatschneider, C., Mercuri-Minich, N. (1994) 'School-age outcomes in children with birth weights under 750 g.' *New England Journal of Medicine*, **331**, 753—759.

Harris, S.R. (1993) 'Evaluating the effects of early intervention. A mismatch between process and product.' *American Journal of Diseases of Children*, **147**, 12–13.

Horn, E.M., Warren, S.F., Jones, H.A. (1995) 'An experimental analysis of a neurobehavioral motor intervention.' *Developmental Medicine and Child Neurology*, **37**, 697–714.

Hughes, I., Newton, R. (1992) 'Genetic aspects of cerebral palsy.' *Developmental Medicine and Child Neurology*, **34**, 80–86.

Hurley, A., Sovner, R. (1987) 'Psychiatric aspects of cerebral palsy.' *Psychiatric Aspects of Mental Retardation Reviews*, **6**, 1–6.

Kohn, J.G. (1990) ' Issues in the management of children with spastic cerebral palsy.' *Pediatrician*, **17**, 230–236.

Kuban, K.C.K., Leviton, A. (1994) 'Cerebral palsy.' *New England Journal of Medicine*, **330**,188–194.

Levitt, S. (1995) *The Treatment of Cerebral Palsy and Motor Delay*. Oxford: Blackwell Scientific.

Little, W.J. (1861–62) 'On the influence of abnormal parturition, difficult labor, premature birth, and asphyxia neonatorum, on the mental and physical condition of the child, especially in relation to deformities.' *Transactions of the Obstetrical Society of London*, **3**, 293–344.

Mac Keith, R. (1976) 'The restoration of the parents as the keystone of the therapeutic arch.' *Developmental Medicine and Child Neurology*, **18**, 285–286. *(Editorial.)*

McCormick, M.C., McCarton, C., Tonascia, J., Brooks-Gunn, J. (1993) 'Early educational intervention for very low birth weight infants: results from the Infant Health and Development Program.' *Journal of Pediatrics*, **123**, 527–533.

McDermott, S., Coker, A.L., Mani, S., Krishnaswami, S., Nagle, R.J., Barnett-Queen, L.L., Wuori, D.F. (1996) 'A population-based analysis of behavior problems in children with cerebral palsy.' *Journal of Pediatric Psychology*, **21**, 447–463.

McGee, J.J. (1988) 'Issues related to applied behavioral analysis.' *In:* Stark, J.A., Menolascino, F.J., Albarelli, M.H., Gray, V.C. (Eds.) *Mental Retardation and Mental Health: Classification, Diagnosis, Treatment, Services*. New York: Springer Verlag, pp. 203–212.

Miller, F., Bachrach, S.J., Duffy, L., Boos, M.L., Pearson, D.T., Walter, R.S., Whinston, J.L. (1995) *Cerebral Palsy: a Complete Guide for Caregiving*. Baltimore: Johns Hopkins University Press.

Minear, W. (1956) 'A classification of cerebral palsy.' *Pediatrics*, **18**, 841.

Mutch, L., Alberman, E., Hagberg, B., Kodama, K., Perat, M.V. (1992) 'Cerebral palsy epidemiology: where are we now and where are we going?' *Developmental Medicine and Child Neurology*, **34**, 547–551.

Naeye, R.L., Peters, E.C., Bartholomew, M., Landis, R. (1989) 'Origins of cerebral palsy.' *American Journal of Diseases of Children*, **143**, 1154–1161.

Nelson, K.B. (1988) 'What proportion of cerebral palsy is related to birth anoxia?' *Journal of Pediatrics*, **112**, 572–574.

——— Ellenberg, J. (1986) 'Antecedents of cerebral palsy.' *New England Journal of Medicine*, **315**, 81–86.

Osler, W. (1889) *The Cerebral Palsies of Children*. (Reprinted 1990 as *Classics in Developmental Medicine No. 1*. London: Mac Keith Press.)

Palisano, R., Rosenbaum, P., Walter, S., Russell, D., Wood, E., Galuppi, B. (1997) 'Development and reliability of a system to classify gross motor function in children with cerebral palsy.' *Developmental Medicine and Child Neurology*, **39**, 214–223.

Palmer, F.B., Shapiro, B.K., Wachtel, R.C., Allen, M.C., Hiller, J.E., Harryman, M.S., Mosher, B.S., Meinert, C.L., Capute, A.J. (1988) 'The effects of physical therapy on cerebral palsy.' *New England Journal of Medicine*, **318**, 803–808.

150

Powell, T.G., Pharoah, P.O.D., Cooke, R.W.I., Rosenbloom, L. (1988a) 'Cerebral palsy in low-birthweight infants. I. Spastic hemiplegia: associations with intrapartum stress.' *Developmental Medicine and Child Neurology*, **30**, 11–18.

—— —— —— —— (1988b) 'Cerebral palsy in low-birthweight infants. II. Spastic diplegia: associations with fetal immaturity.' *Developmental Medicine and Child Neurology*, **30**, 19–25.

Richmond, J.B. (1972) 'The family and the handicapped child.' *Clinical Proceedings of the Children's Hospital National Medical Center*, **8**, 156–64.

Rumeau-Rouquette. C., du Mazaubrun, C., Mlika, A., Dequae, L. (1992) 'Motor disability in children in three birth cohorts.' *International Journal of Epidemiology*, **21**, 359–366.

Rutter, M., Graham, P., Yule, W.A. (1970) *A Neuropsychiatric Study in Childhood. Clinics in Developmental Medicine No. 35/36.* London: Spastics International Medical Publications.

Stanley, F. (1987) 'The changing face of cerebral palsy?' *Developmental Medicine and Child Neurology*, **29**, 263–265.

—— Alberman, E. (1984) *The Epidemiology of the Cerebral Palsies. Clinics in Developmental Medicine No. 87.* Oxford: Blackwell Scientific.

Volpe, J.J. (1992) 'Value of MR in definition of the neuropathology of cerebral palsy in vivo.' *American Journal of Neuroradiology*, **13**, 79–83.

WHO (1980) *International Classification of Impairments, Disabilities, and Handicaps.* Geneva: World Health Organization.

151

INDEX

(Page numbers in *italics* refer to figures/tables.)

A

ABC notation, viii, ix, 79
  autism, 57
abuse
  physical, 12
  sensory impairment, 132
  see also sexual abuse
abusive language, 63, 64
acculturation programmes, 124
Achenback Child Behavior Checklist, 36
achievement, scholastic, 2
activities, meaningful, 129
adoptees, antisocial behaviour, 4, 5
aggression, 1
  function, 58
aggressive behaviour, 7
aggressive interaction with peers, 37
alcoholism, parental, 6
alexithymia, 14
American Sign Language, 95
antisocial behaviour, 1
anxiety, language use in autism, 64, 65
appreciation of child, 14
approval, showing, 80
assistance seeking, 106
ataxia, 138
athetosis in cerebral palsy, 137, 138, 145
attachment relationships, 142
attention, 30
  communicative partners, 104
  gaining in conduct disorder, 15
  joint, 104
  measures, 53
  neuropsychological assessment, 53
  rule, 5
  sustained, 30
attention deficit disorder, deafness, 121
attention deficit–hyperactivity disorder (ADHD), 3,
    28–29
  adulthood, 33
  age of onset, 32
  assessment, 33–38
  behavioural approaches, 40–41
  behavioural management techniques for teachers,
    44
  behavioural observation, 37–38
  behavioural treatment, 38–39
  child interview, 35

clinical diagnosis, 29–30
clinical interview, 34–35
cognitive–behavioural approach, 40–41
cognitive–behavioural training, 45–46
diagnosis, 37
direct interventions, 45–48
DSM-IV, 29, 32
educational modifications, 43–44
environmental interventions, 40
epidemiology, 31–33
learning disorders, 37
mental age assessment, 37
multimodal treatment, 38–41
neuropsychological assessment, 37
noncompliance, 32
nutritional interventions, 39
oppositionality, 32
outcome, 33
overactivity, 31
parent education, 41
parent–child interactions, 38
parenting skills programmes, 42–43
peer interactions, 46
peer problems, 33
positive strategies, 43
prepotent response inhibition, 31
prevalence, 31, 32
psychological testing, 36–37
psychopharmacological interventions, 38, 39–40
punishment, 43
questionnaires, 35–36
rating scales, 35–36
school performance, 32–33
self-esteem, 41
self-image of child, 35
social skills development, 46
teacher feedback, 35
token economies, 43
treatment, 38–48
see also hyperactivity
auditory integration, 70
auditory/oral communication, 123
autism, 54–55
  age at diagnosis, 73
  anxiety, 63, 64, 65
  behaviour
    functional analysis, 58–59
    modification, 67–70
    pattern breaking, 68–69
    rigidity of pattern, 65–66

ritualistic/stereotyped, 67–70
behavioural problems, 55
behavioural variables, 57–58
challenging behaviours, 55, 58–59, 73–74
cognitive assessment, 57
communication, 73–74
    alternative system, 59–60
    impairment, 59–65
    improvement in children who can talk, 61–62
    strategies, 73
computerized communication devices, 61
coping with change, 69
diagnostic features, 56
early behavioural intervention, 68
educational integration, 70
educational placement, 72
emotional problems, 73
environmental factor assessment, 557
environmental modifications, 69
establishment of rules, 68
family needs, 72
goal setting, 68
home-based programmes, 54–55
impairments, vii
intensive behavioural programmes, 70
intervention programmes, 54
joint attention establishment, 104
language
    abstract, 62
    adult, 64
    programmes, 54
mind-reading, 67
obsession use, 69–70
older child, 73
peer relationships, 66–67
pharmacological treatment, 71–72
pictorial communication system, 60–61
provocative speech, 63–64
questioning, 63
reinforcers, viii
repetitive speech, 62–64
respite care, 72
school-based programmes, 55
self-injury, 58
signing, 60
social difficulty amelioration, 65–67
social inhibition lack, 65
social integration, 70
social skills groups, 66
speech development, 59–60
stereotyped behaviours, 67–70
stereotyped speech, 62–64
visual impairment, 131
autistic spectrum disorders, 4
    parenting difficulty, 12
aversives, viii

avoidance–prevention tactic, 89
avoiding trouble, strategies for, 16–21

B
badness of child, pervasive belief, 11
behaviour
    acceptable patterns in autistic children, 65–66
    aggressive, 7
    antisocial, 1
    defining, viii
    differential reinforcement of incompatible, 89–90
    disruptive, 58
    encouraging, 80–84
        learning disabilities, 89–93
    enhancement procedures in cerebral palsy, 147
    fading, 79–80
    high-frequency, 80–81
    ignoring, 16
    impulse, 31
    inappropriate, 87–89, 95–96
    inattentive, 30
    modification
        blindness, 130
        conduct disorder, 21
    prosocial, 38
    school as predictor of adult outcome, 22
    shaping desirable, 16
    written record, 79
    see also challenging behaviour; reinforcers;
        stereotyped behaviours; undesirable behavi-
        ours
behavioural inhibition, cognitive processes, 31
behavioural interventions, cerebral palsy, 146–148
behavioural management techniques for teachers of
    ADHD pupils, 44–45
behavioural problems
    cerebral palsy, 140, 141, 142–143
    sensory impairment, 131–132
behavioural programmes, early intensive for autism,
    70
behavioural therapy, cerebral palsy, 149
biting, reflexive, 146
blindness, 114
    assessment, 115
        behaviour modification, 130
    communication, 119–120, 126
    congenital, 126
    mouthing, 130
    play, 127–128
    residential schools, 123
    stereotyped behaviours, 129–130, 131
    see also visual impairment
bonding, 114
boundaries, conduct disorder, 9
brain
    basal ganglia damage, 138

imaging in cerebral palsy, 142
injury and parenting difficulty, 12

C
cerebral palsy, 136–137
    academic problems, 141
    acquired, 137
    adaptation problems of child, 144–145
    adjustment problems, 144
    assessment, 141–142
    associated disabling conditions, 140–141
    athetosis, 137, 138, 145
    attachment relationships, 142
    authoritarian approach, 147
    behaviour enhancement procedures, 147
    behavioural interventions, 146–148
    behavioural problems, 140, 141, 142–143
    behavioural therapy, 149
    brain
        basal ganglia damage, 138
        damage, 145
        imaging, 142
    causes, 137
    challenging behaviours, 143
    change over time, 139–140
    choreoathetoid, 138, 141
    classification, 136, 138–139
    cognitive impairment, 140
    communication disorders, 140, 142
    denial, 143
    diagnosis, 143
    drug treatment, 149
    dystonia, 138, 140
    environmental stressors, 141
    epilepsy, 141
    family
        adaptation to disability, 143, 144
        history, 143
    growth arrest, 141
    guilt, 143, 145
    impairments, vii
    incidence, 137
    incontinence, 146
    intellectual disability, 141
    interventions, 136
    interviewing child, 144
    learning disabilities, 138
    limb involvement, 139
    management programme, 146–149
    mechanistic attitude, 147
    mental retardation, 141
    mood disorder, 145, 146
    motor disability, 140, 144
    motor function, 139
    motor habilitation, 148
    movement disorder, 136–137, 138

    natural history, 139
    neurodevelopmental examination, 141
    nonspastic types, 138
    outcome, 139
    overprotection, 145, 147
    parent–child relationship, 142
    parents, 143–144, 149
        education, 146
    psychiatric disorders, 141, 145
    psychological attunement, 142
    psychotherapy, 148
    reading difficulties, 141
    relationship models, 142
    schizophrenia, 145
    seizures, 141
    self-blame, 143
    sensory impairment, 141
    social isolation, 143
    social stigma, 145
    spastic types, 137, 138–139
    speech disability, 140, 141
    strabismus, 141
    survival rate, 137
    therapeutic approaches to parents, 148
    tongue thrust, 146
chaining, learning disabilities, 87
challenging behaviour
    autism, 55, 58–59, 73–74
    cerebral palsy, 143
    communication, 59
    function, 58
    learning disabilities, 7
    parenting difficulty, 12
Child and Adolescent Mental Health Services, 20–21
child management, parent training, 41–42
choice making, 107, *108*
chorea, 138
clomipramine, 72
clonidine, 72
cochlear implants, 124
cognitive–behavioural skills in ADHD, 40–41
cognitive–behavioural training in ADHD, 45–46
cognitive impairment in cerebral palsy, 140
cognitive level of function in autism, 57
cognitive processes in conduct disorder, 7
commands, conduct disorder, 15
commenting, topic continuation, 109
commitments, parenting difficulty, 12
communication, 95–96
    assessment, 111
        guidelines, 101–103
    assistance seeking, 106
    augmentative, 62
    autism, 73–74
        impairment, *56*, 59–65

blindness, 119–120, 126
cerebral palsy, 142
challenging behaviour, 59
child input opportunity, 104–105
competence, 96
computerized devices in autism, 61
content, 96
criterion-referenced testing, 101
cultural base, 111
curriculum-referenced testing, 102
deafness, 120, 123–126
delays, 97
development, 110
devices, 146
direct assist strategies, 106–107, *108*, 109–110
disorders, 97
   cerebral palsy, 140
evaluation, 102–103
facilitated, 70
facilitative instructional environment, 105–106
family, 97, *98*
   perception of child's skills, 102
functional, viii
improvement in children who can talk, 61–62
inappropriate behaviour, 95–96
intentional forgetting, 106
intervention, 97, *98*, 102–103
   strategies, 103–107, *108*, 109–110, 110, 111
joint action routines, 106
language
   embedding into daily activities, 105
   interventions, 99
mode for deaf children, 123–126
nonverbal children, 60–61
norm-referenced testing, 101
peer interaction, 105
physical environment, 100
signals, 104
skill
   assessment, 100–103
   facilitation, 98–100
   teaching, 98
social base, 110–111
social communicative context, 103–106
social context, 97, 98
speech, 95
storage of preferred items, 105–106
strategies in autism, 73
success, 96
time delay procedure, 99, *107*, *108*, 110
total, 123, 125
unbiased information in deafness, 125
use, 110
visual impairment, 119–120
wait-time, 104–105
communicative acts, interpretation, 104

communicative independence
   continuum of adult support, *106*
   foundation, 103
   peer interaction opportunities, 105
   promotion, 103
communicative partner
   attention, 104
   skill assessment, 100–101
communicative style, 101
community-based programmes in conduct disorder, 23
computerized communication devices in autism, 61
conduct disorder, 1
   adult outcome, 23
   aetiology, 4–7
   assessment of child, 7–8
   associated features, 1–3
   characteristics of child, 7
   conduct symptoms, 7
   continuity with delinquency, 23
   definition, 1
   desired behaviour increase techniques, 13–15
   differential diagnosis, 3–4
   intervention delivery, 19–21
   learning disabilities, 7
   outcome/outcome predictors, 23–24
   parenting
      assessment, 8–10
      difficulty, 10–12
      programmes, 12–21
   physical examination of child, 8
   poor progress, 18–19
   presentation, 1–4
   prevalence, 4
   prognosis, 23–24
   school information, 8
   school-based programmes, 22–23
   seeing child alone, 7–8
   social impairment, 23
   socialized type, 3
   treatment provision, 20–23
   unsocialized type, 3
conduct problems, parent training programmes, 21
conductive education, vii
Conners rating scales, 36
constitution in conduct disorder, 7
continuous performance test, 53
conversation
   interactions, 109
   response to attempts, 105
   turn-taking, 104, 110
criminality, parental, 6
cultural variants, 4

D
Daily Life Therapy, 71

deaf community, 123, 124
deafness, 114
  action coordination, 120
  attention deficit disorder, 121
  communication, 120
    mode, 123–126
  cultural integration, 126
  language, 120–121
  oral-only communication, 124–125
  parental decisions, 123–124
  play, 128
  postlingual, 124
  residential schools, 123
  social maladjustment, 131
  stereotyped behaviours, 130
  symbolic representation of experiences, 131–132
  testing, 115–116
  see also hearing impairment; sign language;
    signing
defiance, 1
delinquency
  conduct disorder continuity, 23
  well-adjusted, 3
denial
  cerebral palsy, 143
  parental, 117
depression
  parental in conduct disorder, 6
  parenting difficulty, 11
deviance, subcultural, 4
dextroamphetamine, 40
diet
  conduct disorder/hyperactivity, 22
  Feingold, 39
  see also food
differential reinforcement
  of appropriate/alternative behaviour, 147
  of incompatible behaviour, 89–90, 147
  of other behaviours, 147
direct assist strategies
  choice making, 107, *108*
  communication, 106–107, *108*, 109–110
  incidental teaching, *107*, *108*, 110
  mand model, *107*, *108*, 109
  time delay, *107*, *108*, 110
  topic continuation, *107*, *108*, 109–110
discipline in conduct disorder, 9
disobedience, consequences in conduct disorder,
  15–16
disruptive behaviour, function, 58
distraction, 16
drug abuse, 6
drug treatment
  autism, 71–72
  cerebral palsy, 149
  conduct disorder, 22

hyperactivity, 22
  stimulants for ADHD, 39–40
DSM-IV (American Psychiatric Association), 1
  ADHD, 29, 32
  conduct disorder criteria, *2*
  oppositional defiant disorder criteria, *2*
dyslexia, 8
  hyperkinetic disorder, 48
  see also reading difficulties
dystonia, 138

E
echolalia, 62–63
education
  ADHD, 43–44
  see also school
educational placement in autism, 72
emotional abuse, parenting difficulty, 11
emotional attunement/availability of parent in conduct disorder, 9
emotional problems in autism, 73
emotional states, labelling, 14
emotional symptoms in conduct disorder, 1–2
enforcement consistency, 16
environment
  encouraging exploration, 118–120
  facilitative instructional, 105–106
  family, in conduct disorder, 4–5
environmental factor assessment in autism, 55–57
epilepsy in cerebral palsy, 141
expectations, unrealistic, 4, 11
exploration, visual impairment, 119
external stressor, adjustment reaction, 3
extinction
  burst, 64
  reinforcement deprivation, 91
  undesirable behaviours, 91

F
facilitative instructional environment, creation,
  105–106
family
  adaptation to disability in cerebral palsy, 143,
    144
  communication, 97, *98*
  counselling in conduct disorder, 21
  environment in conduct disorder, 4–5
  needs in autism, 72
  perceptions of child's communication skills, 102
Feingold diet, 39
fenfluramine, 71, 72
fining, learning disabilities, 83
fluoxetine, 71
fluvoxamine, 71
food
  allergy and hyperactivity, 39

reinforcers of behaviour, 84
  see also diet
Freedom from Distractability, factor score, 37
functional communication, viii

G

generalized learning disability, 8
  parenting difficulty, 12
genetic predisposition to conduct disorder, 4
gestures, sensory impairment, 125
grief, parental, 117
group work in conduct disorder, 19
growth arrest in cerebral palsy, 141
guilt in cerebral palsy, 143, 145

H

haloperidol, 72
hearing impairment
  development assessment, 115–116
  diagnosis, 115
  language delay, 116
  psychiatric disorders, 131
  social play, 126–127
  see also deafness
heterotypic continuity, conduct disorder, 23
holding therapy, vii, 70
Home Situations Questionnaire, 36
homotypic continuity, conduct disorder, 23
hyperactivity, 3, 28
  age of onset, 32
  assessment, 34–38
  associated difficulties, 32–33
  attention, 30
  behavioural observation, 37–38
  clinical interview, 34–35
  conduct disorder, 1, 2, *3*
  developmental risk factor, 28–29
  diet, 22
  distinction from ADHD, 29
  epidemiology, 31–33
  food allergy, 39
  impairment level, 35
  impulsiveness, 30–31
  learning difficulties, 33
  management in school, 44–45
  medication, 22
  nutritional interventions, 39
  parent training in child management, 41–42
  parenting difficulty, 12
  prevalence, 31, 32
  questionnaires, 8
  school information, 8
  token economies, 43
  treatment plans, 38
  see also attention deficit–hyperactivity disorder
    (ADHD)

hyperkinetic disorder
  case study, 47–48
  clinical diagnosis, 29–30
  diagnosis, 37
  ICD-10 (WHO), 29
  prevalence, 31, 32
hypotonia, early infantile, 140

I

ICD-10 (WHO), 1
  conduct disorder, 1, 3
  hyperkinetic disorder, 29
identity preservation, 114
ignoring behaviour, 16
illness, physical, 12
impulse behaviour, functionality, 31
impulsivity, 30–31
  hyperactivity, 30
  neuropsychological assessment, 53
  targeting in ADHD, 40–41
inappropriate behaviour, 87–89
  communication, 95–96
inattentive behaviour, 30
incontinence, 146
intellectual disability in cerebral palsy, 141
interaction patterns in conduct disorder, 5
interference control, 31
interparental inconsistency, 18
interpreters, 115–116
intervention programmes, vii
interventions, range required, ix
IQ, conduct disorder, 2
isolation, parenting difficulty, 11–12

J

joint action routines in communication, 106
juvenile delinquents, 23
  well-adjusted, 3

L

language
  abstract, 62
  abusive, 63, 64
  adults to autistic children, 64
  assessment guidelines, 101–103
  blindness, 125, 126
  choice making, 107
  deafness, 120–121, 125–126
  delay in hearing impairment, 116
  development, 125–126
  disorders, 95–96
  embedding into daily activities, 105
  environment, 97
  goals, 106, 107
  interventions, 99–100
  naturalistic strategies, 98–99

programmes in autism, 54
skill assessment, 100–103
see also sign language
learning deficit, conduct disorder, 2
learning difficulties
    behaviour in school, 23
    hyperactivity, 33
    school information, 8
learning disabilities
    behaviours, 78–80
        aggressive, 7
        challenging, 7
        encouraging, 80–84, 89–93
        undesirable/inappropriate, 87–89
            not encouraging, 90–91
    cerebral palsy, 138
    chaining, 87
    conduct disorder, 7
    fining, 83
    generalized, 8, 12
    medical screening, 57
    profound, viii
    prompts, 85–86
    reinforcers of behaviour, viii, 80–84
        adapting programme, 82–83
        back-up, 82
        ending programmes, 83–84
    shaping, 85
    star charts, 81–82
    stimulus control, 93
    task analysis, 87
    teaching methods, 84–87
    time out from positive reinforcement, 92
    token programmes, 81–82
learning disorders, ADHD, 37
learning environment assessment, 100
lifestyle, chaotic, 19
linguistic level of function in autism, 57
lip-reading skills, 124
listening skills, 124
lithium, 22

M
Makaton system, 60, 88
maltreatment in sensory impairment, 132
mand model, 99, *107*, *108*, 109
Matching Familiar Figures Test, 53
medication, *see* drug treatment
mental retardation, *see* learning disabilities, gener-
    alized
methylphenidate, 39–40, 47
mind-reading in autism, 67
Monetary Time Sampling, 79
mood disorder in cerebral palsy, 145, 146
morphology, 95
Motivation Assessment Scale, 59

motor disability in cerebral palsy, 140, 144
motor habilitation in cerebral palsy, 148
mouthing, blindness, 130
music therapy, 70
mutual habilitation, 114

N
naltrexone, 72
naturalistic teaching, sensory impairment, 128–129
negotiation in conduct disorder, 17
neighbourhood, 6
neuropsychological assessment, 53
noncompliance, ADHD, 32
nutritional interventions
    ADHD, 39
    see also diet; food

O
obsessions, autism, *56*
off-task behaviours, 37–38
oppositional defiant disorder, 1, *2*
oppositionality in ADHD, 32
Options method for autism, 71
oral-only communication, 124–125
overactivity, 31
overprotection in cerebral palsy, 145, 147

P
paper and pencil cancellation tests, 53
parent–child interactions, conduct disorder, 4–5
parental interview, ADHD, 34–35
parenthood, 114
parenting
    behaviourally based programmes, 12–21
    dimensions, 9–10
    patterns, 10
parenting in conduct disorder, 6
    assessment, 8–10
    poor progress, 18–19
parenting difficulty
    generalized learning disability, 12
    hyperactivity, 12
    intellectual capacity, 11
    isolation, 11–12
    own upbringing, 10–11
    underlying causes, 10–12
    unsupportive partner, 11
parenting skills
    poor progress in conduct disorder, 18–19
    programmes for ADHD, 42–43
parents
    alcoholism, 6
    cerebral palsy, 143–144, 149
    child's needs in conduct disorder, 10
    criminality, 6
    decisions for deaf children, 123–124

depression, 6, 11
education in ADHD/hyperactivity, 41
engaging by clinician, 20
grief, 117
inconsistency, 18
involvement/stimulation in conduct disorder, 9–10
language choice for deaf child, 123–124
positive behaviour, 5
psychiatric disorders/psychosis, 6
therapeutic approaches in cerebral palsy, 148
training
    child management, 41–42
    programmes for conduct problems, 21
peer interaction
    ADHD, 33, 46
    aggressive, 37
    communication, 105
    facilitating, 105
peer relationships
    autism, 66–67
    conduct disorder, 3, 6
perceptual integrity, 114
personality, conduct disorder, 7
phonology, 95
physical abuse, 12
physical care, conduct disorder, 10
physical factor assessment in autism, 55–57
Picture Exchange Communication System, 60–61, 95
pictures, undesirable behaviour avoidance, 88
play
    blindness, 127–128
    deafness, 128
    intervenors for sensory impaired children, 128
    parenting programmes for conduct disorder, 13–14
    sensory impairment, 122
    social, 126–127
pragmatics, 95
Pragmatics Profile of Early Communication Skills, 62
praise in conduct disorder, 14–15
Premack Principle, 80
prepotent response inhibition, 31
preschool education for disadvantaged children, 23
problem-solving approach to conduct disorder, 17
    skills training, 21–22
Project ECLIPSE curriculum, 103
prompts in learning disabilities, 85–86
prosocial behaviours, 38
provocative speech, 63–64
psychiatric disorders
    cerebral palsy, 141, 145
    parenting difficulty, 11
    sensory impairment, 131

psychological attunement in cerebral palsy, 142
psychological testing, 36–37
psychopathology screening, 36
psychosis, parental, 6
psychotherapy
    cerebral palsy, 148
    individual in conduct disorder, 22
punishment, 43

Q

questioning
    repetitive, 63
    stimulus control, 93
    topic continuation, 109
questionnaires
    ADHD, 35–36
    hyperactivity, 8

R

rating scales, ADHD, 35–36
reading difficulties, 2
    ADHD, 32–33
    cerebral palsy, 141
    see also dyslexia
rehabilitation, 114
reinforcers, viii
    backup, 82
    facilitative instructional environment, 105
    food, 84
    inadvertant, 90–91
    learning disabilities, 80–84
    social, 92
    token economies, 43
    see also time out from positive reinforcement
relationships
    difficulties in conduct disorder, 19
    models for cerebral palsy, 142
    parenting difficulty, 11
respite care, autism, 72
response, stopping ongoing, 31
retinopathy of prematurity, 115
rewards, 14
    token economies, 43
Ritalin, see methylphenidate
ritualistic behaviours in autism, 56, 67–70
Rutter scales, 36

S

sanctions, viii
schizophrenia, 145
school
    factors in conduct disorder, 6
    information in conduct disorder, 8
    performance
        ADHD, 32–33
        conduct disorder, 2

159

residential for sensory impaired children, 123
 see also education
School Situations Questionnaire, 36
school-based programmes
 autism, 55
 conduct disorder, 22–23
schooling
 modifications in ADHD, 43–44
 special needs, 22–23
scotopic sensitivity training, 70
script use, topic continuation, 109–110
sedatives, 22
seizures, cerebral palsy, 137, 141
self-blame by parents, 143
self-concept in sensory impairment, 123
self-control targeting in ADHD, 40–41
self-esteem
 stress levels in parents of children with sensory
  impairment, 118
 targeting in ADHD, 41
self-image of child, 35
self-injury
 autism, 58
 function, 58
 physical basis of behaviour, 57
self-talk strategies, 45
semantics, 95
sensory ability, residual, 128
sensory experiences, 114
sensory impairment, 114
 abuse, 132
 behavioural problems, 131–132
 cerebral palsy, 141
 congenital, 132
 contacts with children sharing perceptual differences, 123
 development, assessment, 115–117
 diagnosis, 115
 early intervention, 118–119
 environmental stimulation, 121–122
 gestures, 125
 interpretation of tests, 116–117
 intervenors for play, 128
 interventions for optimum development, 118–132
 maltreatment, 132
 meaningful activity, 129
 multidisciplinary assessment, 117
 naturalistic teaching, 128–129
 object relationships, 120–121
 parental reaction to diagnosis, 117
 parental support, 118
 play, 122
 professional support for family, 117–118
 psychiatric disorders, 131–132
 residual sensory ability, 128
 social interactions, 122–123

social isolation, 132
social play, 126–128
sorting activities, 121
stereotyped behaviours, 129–130, 131
stress levels on parents, 118
suddenly acquired, 132
toys, 121–122
separation anxiety disorder, 145
serotonin uptake inhibitors, 71
sexual abuse
 conduct disorder, 6
 parenting difficulty, 12
shaping, learning disabilities, 85
sign language, 123, 124
 American, 95
 deaness, 115
 family participation, 125
sign system, autism, 60
signals, communication, 104
signing
 deafness, 123
 undesirable behaviour avoidance, 88, 89
social behaviour rules, 66
social difficulty, amelioration in autism, 65–67
social environment, communication, 100
social impairment, conduct disorder, 23
social inhibition, lack in autism, 65
social interactions, sensory impairment, 122–123
social isolation
 cerebral palsy, 143
 sensory impairment, 132
social play, sensory impairment, 126–128
social relationships, conduct disorder, 2–3
social skills
 development in ADHD, 46
 groups for autism, 66
 learning in conduct disorder, 5
 training for conduct disorder, 21–22
social understanding, impairment in autism, *56*
Social Use of Language Programme, 62
social work, conduct disorder, 21
socioeconomic conditions, parenting difficulty, 12
sorting activities, 121
spasticity, 138
 early infantile hypotonia, 140
Special Educational Needs Coordinators, 23
special needs schooling, 22–23
specific reading disorder, 2
speech
 communication, 95
 development in autism, 59–60
 disability in cerebral palsy, 140, 141
 repetitive/stereotyped, 62–64
star charts, 81–82, 83
stereotyped behaviours
 autism, 67–70

blindness, 129–130, 131
  deafness, 130
  function, 58
  sensory impairment, 129–130
stimulant medication, 39–40, 47
stimulus control, 93
strabismus, 141
Strengths and Difficulties Questionnaire, 8, 36
supervision, conduct disorder, 9, 17
support services for sensory impaired children, 117–118
swearing, 63, 64
  reinforcing, 90–91
symbolic representation of experiences of deaf children, 131–132
syntax, 95

T
task analysis, learning disabilities, 87
TEACCH educational programme, 62, 72
teachers
  behavioural management techniques for ADHD, 44–45
  training, 22
teaching
  incidental, *107*, *108*, 110
    for communication, 99
  methods for learning disabilities, 84–87
temperament, conduct disorder, 7
theory of mind, deficits, 67
tics, 40
time delay procedure for communication, 99, *107*, *108*, 110
time out (time out from positive reinforcement), 16
  ADHD, 43
  autism, 55, 64
  cerebral palsy, 147
  conduct disorder, 16
  learning disabilities, 92
token economies, 43
  programmes for learning disabilities, 81–82
tongue thrust, 146
topic continuation, *107*, *108*, 109–110
toys, noise making, 120
tranquillizers, 22
treatment, vii
  ADHD, 34, 38–48
    behavioural, 40–48
    nutritional, 38
    psychopharmacological, 38–40

autism, 70–72
  behavioural, 70, 73
  improving communication skills, 59–65
  pharmacological, 71–72
    vitamin, 71
behaviourally based, vii–viii
cerebral palsy, 136, 146–149
  behavioural/psychological, 146–148
  pharmacological, 149
conduct disorder, 20–23
  behavioural, 12–17
  child-based, 21–22
  community-based, 23
  family, 21
  parental attitude to child, 9
  school-based, 22–23
tricyclic antidepressants, 40

U
understanding impairment in autism, *56*
undesirable behaviours, 87–89
  avoiding action, 89
  extinction, 91
  not encouraging, 90–91
  understanding, 88
upbringing, adverse, 4

V
vision stimulation teachers, 119
visual impairment
  associated impairments, vii
  autism, 131
  communication, 119–120
  diagnosis, 115
  exploration, 119
  interventions for optimum development, 119
  language development, 126
  psychiatric disorders, 131
  touch dependence, 119–120
  toys, 120
  see also blindness
vitamin treatments, autism, 71

W
wait-time, communication, 104–105
Wechsler Intelligence Scale for Children, 37
Wechsler Objective Reading Dimensionstest, 37

X
XYY karyotype, 4

161